HEALTH BEHAVIOR CHANGE AND TREATMENT ADHERENCE

HEALTH BEHAVIOR CHANGE AND TREATMENT ADHERENCE

Evidence-Based Guidelines for Improving Healthcare

Leslie R. Martin
La Sierra University

Kelly B. Haskard-Zolnierek
Texas State University, San Marcos

M. Robin DiMatteo
University of California, Riverside

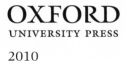

2010

OXFORD
UNIVERSITY PRESS

Oxford University Press, Inc., publishes works that further
Oxford University's objective of excellence
in research, scholarship, and education.

Oxford New York
Auckland Cape Town Dar es Salaam Hong Kong Karachi
Kuala Lumpur Madrid Melbourne Mexico City Nairobi
New Delhi Shanghai Taipei Toronto

With offices in
Argentina Austria Brazil Chile Czech Republic France Greece
Guatemala Hungary Italy Japan Poland Portugal Singapore
South Korea Switzerland Thailand Turkey Ukraine Vietnam

Published by Oxford University Press, Inc.
198 Madison Avenue, New York, New York 10016

www.oup.com

Oxford is a registered trademark of Oxford University Press, Inc.

Library of Congress Cataloging-in-Publication Data
Martin, Leslie R.
Health behavior change and treatment adherence : evidence-based guidelines for improving
healthcare / Leslie R. Martin, Kelly B. Haskard Zolnierek, M. Robin DiMatteo.
p. ; cm.
Includes bibliographical references.
ISBN-13: 978-0-19-538040-8 (alk. paper)
ISBN-10: 0-19-538040-1 (alk. paper)
1. Patient compliance. 2. Health behavior. I. Haskard Zolnierek, Kelly B., 1978–
II. DiMatteo, M. Robin. III. Title.
[DNLM: 1. Health Behavior. 2. Evidence-Based Medicine. 3. Patient Compliance.
W 85 M3815h 2010]
R727.43.M37 2010
613—dc22

2009016643

9 8 7 6 5 4 3 2 1

Printed in the United States of America
on acid-free paper

To my parents, who gave me life and promote my health (LRM)
For Jamie, Kirra, Mom, Dad, and Alec (KBHZ)
For my students at the University of California, Riverside (MRD)

Preface

When we set out to write this book we asked ourselves, "Why is it that changing health behaviors and maintaining good health habits can be so difficult when the behaviors themselves are often quite simple?" Many empirical studies have addressed aspects of this question, but reviewing the thousands of research papers that exist on patient adherence and health behavior change can be daunting. When combined with complementary bodies of research on topics such as persuasion, goal-setting, and motivation, the volume of literature can be, quite simply, overwhelming. Our aim in writing this book has been to distill from these vast bodies of literature some key principles that govern the performance of health behaviors and the most effective strategies that facilitate change and promote adherence.

This volume is designed to be both informative and enjoyable to read; ideally it would be "pleasure-reading" with a very practical purpose! We have written for a broad audience that includes practitioners and students in all areas of medicine including allopathic, osteopathic, and chiropractic, and also for other health professionals such as physician assistants, nurses, dentists, clinical and health psychologists, marriage and family counselors, social workers, school psychologists, and care administrators (e.g., directors of elder care facilities). We also address our book to the layperson who wishes to take an active role in changing his or her health behaviors. In short, this book has been researched and written for anyone who wants to improve their own health and well-being or that of others.

Simple, powerful, and practical strategies are needed to guide individuals who want to change their own behaviors and health professionals who wish to help their clients put long-term health-relevant behavior changes into practice. We advocate for a straightforward "3-component approach": Before a person can change, they must *(1)* know what change is necessary (*information*); *(2)* desire the change (*motivation*); and then *(3)* have the tools to achieve and maintain the change (*strategy*). Information, motivation, and strategy are the essential ingredients, and these are woven throughout this text.

In our book, we first focus on theoretical models of health behavior change, including the factors that influence motivation and the most effective strategies for creating and maintaining desired changes. Next, we investigate the healthcare process itself as a way of understanding and creating effective disease-prevention and management regimens. We pay special attention to the individual's role in creating positive habits, evaluating risks and benefits, and effectively communicating with various healthcare partners. Finally, we tackle issues related to working effectively within the constraints of the healthcare system, including the ways in which technology can be helpful, and the ways in which partnerships between clinicians and their patients (or clients) can help minimize barriers to effective healthcare.

In addition to presenting a timely synthesis of empirically based knowledge across a number of relevant fields of study, we offer succinct, evidence-based recommendations and strategies for implementing the described techniques. We do this because, while many practitioners (and patients) know a great deal about *what* should be done, people generally know very little about *how* to effectively act to achieve health goals. And, although some influences and effects are intuitive (e.g., the relevance of liking, expertise, and persuasion), the extent and direction of the effects (e.g., certain extrinsic motivators) are often unknown or misunderstood. Thus, while some of these strategies may be familiar in name to some people, they tend to be poorly understood, rarely taught, and even less often linked together systematically. We also point out common misconceptions that persist about contemporary healthcare, and in their place we provide information and strategic recommendations grounded in solid research.

We are grateful to those who have encouraged us throughout this process, and to our editor at Oxford University Press, Lori Handelman, who was helpful in ways too many to mention. Robin DiMatteo would also like to acknowledge the Robert Wood Johnson Foundation Investigator Award in Health Policy for continued support of her research on physician-patient communication and disparities in health care (although the views expressed in this book are those of the authors alone, and do not imply endorsement by RWJF). All three of us would like to acknowledge our Psychology Department colleagues at our respective institutions—La Sierra University; Texas State University, San Marcos; and the University of California, Riverside—whose energy, vitality, and commitment to research and teaching continue to inspire and support our work.

Contents

HEALTH BEHAVIOR CHANGE AND TREATMENT ADHERENCE

1

Understanding Behavior Change: The Theory Behind Informing, Motivating, and Planning for Health

Essentially, all models are wrong, but some are useful.
—George Box, Professor Emeritus, University of Wisconsin

Common stereotypes suggest that when it comes to setting goals about lifestyle and health, there are three types of people. Alex is the first type. He is exceedingly competent at setting goals and achieving them. He maintains a fit and healthy body while balancing his career goals with time for his family, friends, hobbies, and contributions to the community. Alex is the person that many of us believe we could be "if only" we would apply ourselves. Others of us, of course, see these behaviors as far beyond the realm of possibility, so far that we don't even consider trying to achieve them. Meg is the second type. She sets goals constantly (for example, losing 10 lbs before the holidays or joining a gym and working out "every day"). Unfortunately, temptations or other barriers often lead to quick failures. Meg follows with yet another set of new goals the next day or next week, only to fail once more. "Life happens" to Meg; in her opinion, little is within her control. We might sympathize with Meg for being disorganized or even lazy. We might feel that she "really ought to be able to change." Perhaps we even feel a bit critical and superior, despite our own difficulties achieving the health goals that we set. Zach is the third type of person. He doesn't even recognize the importance of health behavior change. Zach doesn't worry about being overweight, living a sedentary lifestyle, or continuing to smoke. For Zach, improving health seems like a good idea for other people, but it isn't worth the effort for him.

In reality, very few people are precisely the same as any of these stereotypical individuals. Instead most people fall somewhere in between—demonstrating great competence and success in pursuing some aspects of a healthy lifestyle, but remaining uninformed and unmotivated, or struggling and failing, in others. Most

3

people actually try to make behavioral changes often, but much less frequently are able to maintain them. "Real life" does indeed interfere with people's plans to be healthy. The good news is that there are plenty of opportunities for life's trajectories to be directed and purposeful. Let's explore some of these.

Levels of Health Behavior

There are many ways to promote health and wellness, at various levels, and it makes sense to try to understand these systematically. The type of intervention, and the effectiveness of behavioral efforts in changing actual health status, depends in part on a person's current health status. Health behaviors can thus be categorized according to where in the "disease-risk cycle" they fall. This is done by distinguishing between primary, secondary, and tertiary preventive behaviors.

Primary prevention refers to behaviors that a healthy person enacts in order to maximize well-being and avoid particular diseases.[1] In the previous section, we met Alex, who is fit and seems to have achieved balance in his life. He practices many elements of primary prevention such as power-walking three times per week, continuing to improve his eating habits, and practicing meditation to help manage stress. Alex does not have any diagnosed diseases and is not in any high-risk groups, but this doesn't mean that Alex doesn't need to think about his health. He strives actively to promote good health and to prevent future negative health outcomes.

Secondary prevention describes behaviors that an individual undertakes after a particular risk has been identified. These behaviors are meant to forestall the more serious but likely outcomes that would be the result of continuing "life as usual." Remember Meg? Despite the fact that she tries to change her health behaviors, she is generally unsuccessful. In particular she struggles to resist junk food and her weight is higher than it should be. As a result she has recently been diagnosed with hypertension. So, Meg's physician has prescribed an antihypertensive medication for her to take daily and has recommended that Meg have her blood pressure checked regularly. Meg does not currently have a disease, but her high blood pressure places her at risk for heart disease and stroke, among other problems. Because taking medication and getting blood pressure checks are focused on preventing diseases that could result from hypertension, these behaviors involve secondary prevention. Eating well and exercising are examples of behaviors that can fit into more than one category of prevention, depending on the individual; they are also applicable for Meg in preventing hypertension. What distinguishes them from the primary prevention behaviors of Alex is that Meg currently is *at risk*, whereas Alex is not.

Tertiary prevention behaviors are those that a person undertakes in order to control the progression of a disease, or to cure it. Zach is a smoker. If he were to be diagnosed with lung cancer, he would need to begin a chemotherapy regimen

designed to eradicate the disease from his body. Faithfully meeting his chemotherapy appointments would represent a tertiary prevention behavior, that is,
a behavior designed to prevent the further progression of the disease and eventual
death. As we will see throughout this chapter, the process of changing health
behaviors is complex and varies according to many different factors. The level at
which the health behavior is targeted is one of these factors.

Theoretical Models of Health Behavior and Change

For several decades, both researchers and practitioners in health-related fields
including psychology, public health, medicine, nursing, dentistry, chiropractic,
counseling, and health-care administration, have been trying to understand the
factors that contribute to, or inhibit, an individual's success in achieving and
maintaining health behavior change. These health professionals and researchers
have developed a number of useful theoretical models for understanding what
people believe about health, why they take health actions (or fail to do so), and
how they maintain behavioral change. While some explanatory models have
received more empirical evaluation than others, each can be helpful in some
contexts and can provide a useful organizational structure to help us address the
maintenance of health behavior change and adherence to treatment plans.

Prominent in these models are the constructs of "beliefs" and "attitudes." Beliefs
involve conclusions about the truth of something, and are *cognitive* elements in the
picture of how people evaluate and respond to ideas. Attitudes involve affective
(emotional) elements and involve *evaluative states* based on the individual's personal
feelings and emotions regarding a belief. In other words, attitudes subsume beliefs.
For example, if Zach believes that exercise is unpleasant, his attitude toward exercise
will likely be negative, even if he is willing to admit (i.e., he believes) that exercise is
important.

Two psychologists, Icek Ajzen and Martin Fishbein, first proposed in the 1970s
that beliefs precede attitudes, and further that attitudes are the precursors for (and
driving forces behind) individuals' intentions to perform behavior as well as their
actual performance.[2] Others have built upon these foundational ideas, and below
we examine the best-known models of health behavior along with the contributions
they have made to our understanding of behavior change and adherence. We
provide explanations of how each model has most often and most effectively been
used, as well as a summary of problems or weaknesses in each of the approaches.

Health Belief Model

The Health Belief Model was originally developed to explain when people
would (and would not) engage in preventive health behaviors.[3] In the early
1950s, researchers at the U.S. Public Health Service were specifically

interested in why some people with no symptoms underwent x-ray screening for tuberculosis while others would refuse to obtain needed immunizations. More research studies have been based on this model than on any other. The Health Belief Model focuses primarily on beliefs as the motivators of health behavior. These include: *(1)* beliefs about how susceptible or at-risk a person is to a particular disease or other negative health outcome, *(2)* beliefs about how severe an illness or negative health outcome might be, if the person did develop it, *(3)* beliefs about whether recommended treatments are effective or whether health behavior change is feasible and beneficial, and *(4)* beliefs about how well-equipped one is to confront the challenges of achieving and maintaining health. These challenges include such potential barriers as the inability to regulate one's own behavior, the financial cost associated with treatment, and the time constraints of health behavior.

Additional factors that have been added to the model over the years include demographic characteristics (e.g., age, gender) and environmental cues (e.g., a doctor's recommendation, a friend's heart attack) that might motivate a person to take action.[4] These additions highlight the fact that while individual perceptions, beliefs, and attitudes are critically important, they are not sufficient to predict actual health behaviors. One must look to the individual's life to understand the role of other idiosyncratic factors as well.

As with all health behavior and change models, the Health Belief Model has some limitations. Over the years, for example, some elements have been added to the original Health Belief model, although in research studies they have not always been well measured, have sometimes been only loosely connected to underlying theory, or have failed to demonstrate good empirical links with behavioral outcomes. And, some research on the model has focused on the outcome of behavioral *intentions* rather than on actual behaviors. This has led to some murkiness when trying to evaluate the utility of the Health Belief Model as a template for designing effective health behavior interventions. Nonetheless, the Health Belief Model is one of the best known health behavior theories and it makes important contributions to understanding health behavior. This is true particularly because the Health Belief Model emphasizes the crucial role of an individual's *perceptions* when it comes to choosing and carrying out his or her health behaviors.

After 1988, self-efficacy (the belief that one is capable of enacting change) was formally added to the Health Belief Model, making an important, though modest, contribution to the ability of this model to predict behavioral outcomes.[5] Incorporating efficacy expectations into the model along with expectations for what will happen following a behavior (outcome expectancies) suggests additional ways in which the model might be used to develop effective interventions for helping people to change their health behaviors. Recent research applications of the Health Belief Model show that addressing people's efficacy expectations—their belief in their ability to change—can help to enhance the effect of health beliefs in changing health behaviors.

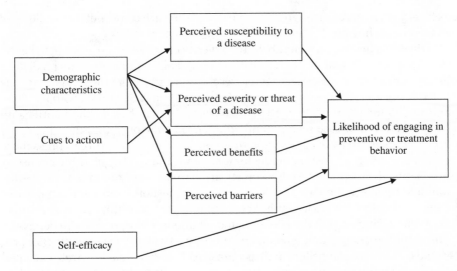

Figure 1.1 Health belief model.

The body of research involving the Health Belief Model has become quite substantial. In 1984, Janz and Becker reviewed 46 studies conducted between 1956 and 1984.[6] Twenty-four of these focused on preventive health behaviors (e.g., immunizations, screenings, exercise), 19 on behaviors related to the sick role (e.g., adherence to treatment regimens, seeing a physician for symptoms), and three on clinic utilization (e.g., clinic visits, appointment-keeping). Each of the dimensions of the Health Belief Model was significantly associated with health behavior and change. Of the various elements of the model, peoples' perceptions of the barriers to change figured most importantly in predicting actual health behavior. Barriers were followed closely by perceived susceptibility, perceived benefits associated with change, and finally perceived severity of the disease or other negative health outcome. It has been hypothesized that perceptions of disease severity might be relatively less important to individuals who are contemplating primary prevention behaviors and more important to those who already have a diagnosis and want to prevent disease progression.

More recent studies of the Health Belief Model are generally consistent with findings from the 1984 large-scale review study, and show that the elements of the HBM can be ordered in terms of their importance in predicting change. For instance, Wallace's study of college women's engagement in weight-bearing exercise and intake of calcium to prevent osteoporosis found that self-efficacy, perceived barriers, and perceived susceptibility were the strongest predictors of these health actions.[7] Another recent study of the expanded Health Belief Model examined the frequency of individual diabetes management behaviors (e.g., exercise, diet, blood sugar testing, insulin injections, etc.) and demonstrated that perceived barriers and self-efficacy were most strongly associated with a variety of individual diabetes management behaviors.[8]

In these studies, perceptions about the severity of a disease do not seem to be the most important element of the Health Belief Model's contribution to predicting behavior, but in some cases severity perceptions are still quite meaningful. Beliefs about severity appear to play a larger role for those already diagnosed with a disease than they do for primary prevention. A recent meta-analysis of the relationship between perceived disease severity and adherence behaviors found that if patients believe that their disease is serious and threatening, they are almost 2.5 times more likely to adhere to their treatment recommendations than if they view the disease as less ominous.[9] (A meta-analysis is a statistical technique used to combine the results of multiple studies that address the same research question.) Table 1.1 summarizes this meta-analysis, along with other key meta-analyses of health behavior change. These findings suggest that the adoption and maintenance of good health behaviors require health messages and recommendations, particularly from health-care professionals, that are compelling and persuasive. If individuals are well educated about the potential dangers of unhealthy behavior and the diseases those behaviors might cause, they are more likely to follow recommendations for health behavior change.

Theory of Reasoned Action

The idea that people's behaviors are primarily governed by their *intentions*, which in turn spring from a combination of their attitudes toward and social norms regarding those behaviors, was formalized in the mid- to late 1970s.[2, 10] According to this formulation, attitudes involve an overlay of feeling and emotion on specific beliefs that the individual holds. When this idea was first proposed, however, it represented a distinct divergence from earlier social psychological thought, which viewed attitudes as a "readiness" to respond in a particular way to environmental stimuli. Many studies had demonstrated, however, that attitudes were not always very closely related to actual behaviors. These findings necessitated the development of a more complex model to explain the attitude-behavior relationship, and the Theory of Reasoned Action was born.

Two elements of the Theory of Reasoned Action are particularly noteworthy. The first is that changes in belief are necessary to effect changes in behavior because all behavioral choices are ultimately based on beliefs of one sort or another. Second, an individual's behavioral intention (which is the best predictor of the behavior itself) is governed by the relative importance of his or her personal *attitudes* toward the behavior and *subjective norms* (that is, the person's beliefs about what others think about the behavior and whether the person *cares* what others think).

Thus, for any specific behavior, personal attitudes may be more or less important depending on the weight carried by the subjective norms. Zach's attitude

Table 1.1 Summary of selected meta-analyses of key models of health behavior change.

Model	Author	Date	Number of Samples/ Studies	Components of Theory	Outcome Variables	Synopsis of Results
Health Belief Model	Janz & Becker	1984	46 (18 prospective; 28 retrospective)	Perceived susceptibility, severity, benefits, and barriers	Preventive health behaviors, sick role behaviors, clinic utilization	Strongest predictors across study designs and health behaviors (in order): barriers, susceptibility, benefits, and severity
	DiMatteo, Haskard, & Williams	2007	27	Perceived severity	Patient Adherence	Positive relationship between perceived severity and adherence
	Harrison, Mullen, & Green	1992	16	Perceived susceptibility, severity, benefits, and costs	Health behavior	Retrospective studies had larger effects for benefits and costs compared to severity
Theory of Reasoned Action	Sheppard, Hartwick, & Warshaw	1988	174	Intentions and Behavior (I-B); Attitudes + Subjective norms and Intentions (A+SN − I)	Goals and Behavior	Model has predictive utility; Three significant moderators: measure of intention; prediction of goals vs. behavior; the choice among various options
Theory of Planned Behavior	Armitage & Connor	2001	185	Attitude, subjective norms, and perceived behavioral control; intentions and behaviors	Observed or self-reported behaviors and intentions	Better predictive utility for self-reported behaviors; strong intention-behavior relationship and perceived behavioral control and behavior relationship; subjective norms weakly related to intentions

(Continued)

Table 1.1 (Continued)

Model	Author	Date	Number of Samples/ Studies	Components of Theory	Outcome Variables	Synopsis of Results
Theory of Reasoned Action and Theory of Planned Behavior	Albarracin, Johnson, Fishbein, & Muellerleile	2001	96	Intentions, attitudes, subjective norms; perceived behavioral control	Condom use	Condom use was significantly associated with intentions, attitudes and subjective norms; perceived behavioral control predicted intentions but did not significantly predict condom use
Social Cognitive Theory*	Holden	1991	56	Self-efficacy	Health outcomes	Ratings of self-efficacy predicted health outcomes
Transtheoretical Model of Change	Marshall & Biddle	2001	91	Precontemplation, Contemplation, Preparation, Action, Maintenance	Exercise and physical activity	Many studies cross-sectional so don't verify the stage theory; there were differences in activity across stage levels and most changes happening at higher order stages
Precaution Adoption Process Model	No meta-analytic reviews					
Information-Motivation-Strategy Model	No meta-analytic reviews					

*Social Cognitive Theory (SCT) relevant, though not a meta-analysis of complete SCT.

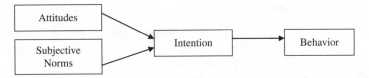

Figure 1.2 Theory of reasoned action.

toward quitting smoking, for example, will be partly determined by his beliefs about the link between smoking and lung cancer but may also be influenced by the opinions of his family and friends. Thus, having a group of close friends who also smoke and who are not willing to quit might make Zach less inclined to commit himself to quitting, even if he personally believes that smoking leads to lung cancer and is worried about this prospect for himself.

According to the Theory of Reasoned Action, effective health behavior interventions will take into account the degree to which a particular behavioral intention is influenced by social norms and personal attitudes. Strategies designed to modify beliefs can then be appropriately targeted to the area that most influences behavior.

A great deal of research has focused on testing the tenets of this model, although in many cases researchers have interpreted the model rather loosely by measuring behavioral outcomes that are not completely under the individual's control, or by assessing and using behavioral predictors while various intentions are still somewhat in flux for the individual. Also, just as with the Health Belief Model, research studies have often used behavioral intentions as the measured outcome, instead of actual behaviors. This is not a significant problem, because intentions are both most proximal to behavior and a necessary precursor to health-related decisions and behaviors. The outcome of behavioral intentions does warrant mention, however, because the focus of the model itself is the explicit prediction of *behavior*. Despite these caveats, the predictive utility of the model is robust across a variety of behavioral outcomes.[11]

One recent meta-analysis of studies on condom use found that this safe sex behavior was related to intentions based on subjective norms and attitudes, and that these attitudes were, in turn, based on normative and behavioral beliefs.[12] Indeed, as predicted by the model, what others did and thought helped influence individuals' own condom use. Another meta-analysis, this one focused on physical activity as the behavioral outcome, confirmed the importance of a person's intentions, as well as the links between intentions, attitudes, and beliefs for predicting an individual's engagement in an activity.[13] In addition to physical activity and safe sex, a wide range of other health behaviors including contraception, sunscreen use, mammography screening, weight loss, smoking cessation, and AIDS risk-related behaviors can be predicted using the Theory of Reasoned Action.[14–18]

Theory of Planned Behavior

The Theory of Planned Behavior is an extension of the Theory of Reasoned Action that was formulated in the 1980s, and is specifically targeted at situations in which individuals do not have full control over the behavior in question.[19, 20] As in the Theory of Reasoned Action, an individual's intention is of central importance, but here it is influenced not only by attitudes and subjective norms but also by perceived behavioral control (which is an individual's belief about the amount of control he or she has over a given behavior). Perceived behavioral control is very similar to the concept of self-efficacy, described as part of the expanded Health Belief Model. Perceived behavioral control involves the individual's confidence that he or she can enact change. This already-complex model is made even more complicated by the fact that the relative importance of each of these three elements (attitudes, subjective norms, perceived behavioral control) varies according to the situation.

This added complexity provides flexibility to the model, increasing our ability to better understand each particular health behavior for a specific person. It also emphasizes how important it is to understand the relative role of each component when attempting to change behavior. Research models cannot be applied to individual people using a simple recipe-book approach, expecting that the outcomes will be equivalent for everyone or across different situations.

As is often true, this model's intricacy makes it a better representation of reality but also makes it more difficult to test. Despite this, a comparison of the Theory of Reasoned Action with the Theory of Planned Behavior has shown that, for a variety of behaviors, the inclusion of perceptions of behavioral control allows for better prediction of both intentions and behaviors, especially when behaviors are clearly under a person's volitional control.[21, 22] Thus, research suggests that an individual is more likely to attempt a behavior if success seems likely. In fact, even when accomplishment of an aim is not clearly under one's control, the *perception that it is* can still be valuable.

A 2001 meta-analysis of 185 studies published between 1985 and 1997 similarly found that including perceived behavioral control improved the predictive

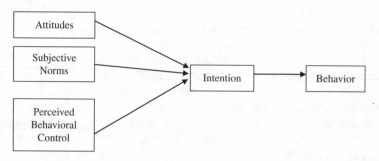

Figure 1.3 Theory of planned behavior.

ability of the model. Furthermore, perceptions of control seem to have influenced intentions because a person's belief that he or she "can do it" typically prompts an individual to make a commitment to try. Perceptions of control are also related to subsequent behaviors because the individual's belief that he or she can accomplish the behavior tends to prompt him or her to actually initiate it once the commitment is made.[23] Thus, for example, if Zach doesn't believe he has the willpower to quit smoking, he is less likely to take on the challenge of trying to quit.

This important meta-analysis also showed that the link between subjective norms and intentions is less robust than are other connections in the model; that is, subjective norms are poorer predictors of behavioral intentions. This raises questions about the way subjective norms are measured. Typically these norms are assessed with a single item and so the link may be weak partly because the measurement is inadequate.

This apparent methodological weakness highlights the importance of examining subjective norms carefully and with powerful assessment tools. For example, it has been suggested that the social pressure of subjective norms is moderated by the degree to which an individual identifies with a group of people whose health behavior is relevant to the individual.[24] A good measurement tool will, therefore, assess not only the norm itself but also the degree to which the individual identifies with those who create the norm. Alex, for example, might identify strongly with his work colleagues who are all committed to maintaining a healthy lifestyle. Alex's identification with his coworkers renders his subjective norms in this area much more powerful than Meg's. Meg's colleagues are also committed to good health, but she doesn't feel she has much in common with them and this weakens their social power in influencing her behavior.

Transtheoretical Model of Change

The Transtheoretical Model grew out of an effort to understand the process of change within a psychotherapeutic setting.[25] In the initial stages of developing of this model, during the late 1970s and early 1980s, several processes of change were defined, including the following. *(1) Consciousness raising*, which involves techniques that are aimed at increasing a person's awareness. In Zach's case, this could involve providing feedback to him about the health risks associated with his smoking. *(2) Choosing among options*, which allows an individual to see or create more options and to take personal responsibility for determining his or her subsequent behavior. And finally, *(3) Contingency control*, which involves providing resources to help a person change their environments and the associated system of rewards and punishments so as to maximize their behavior-change success.

In ongoing work with these concepts, Prochaska and DiClemente suggested that regardless of whether individuals were engaged in psychotherapeutic change or another kind of behavior change they typically seemed to progress through a series of stages.[26] These stages involved first thinking about changing a behavior, then becoming determined to enact the change, then actively modifying their habits or environments, and finally, finding ways to maintain the change. These researchers also found that thinking through and verbalizing different options was especially important when individuals were thinking about and becoming determined to take action. Controlling contingencies seemed not to be used (or to be used ineffectively) until the individual had reached the stage of actively modifying her or his habits.

One very useful aspect of this model (indeed, of change models in general) is the assumption that what will most effectively move a person toward the ultimate behavioral goal may vary depending on the individual's current stage. The best strategies for one stage may not be the most effective techniques at another stage. For instance, when Zach is not giving any serious thought to changing his lifestyle, he is not likely to pay much attention to collaborative efforts to devise a system to reward his good health behaviors. He is also not likely to stick to a behavioral change system if someone else designs it for him. Meg, however, *does* want to change; in fact, she is constantly (though unsuccessfully) attempting to create healthy habits. Because she does care and wants to make changes, she is likely to be motivated to work with a health professional to create a personalized and effective plan. She is also likely to put forth a good effort toward implementing the plan. When a person is trying to change (or to help others change), various tools, interventions, and strategies will be most successful if they are matched to the individual's current location in his or her change process.

The Transtheoretical Model of Change was formalized in 1983 with five stages of change that subsumed ten separate proposed processes for change.[27] These five stages were later revised (based on reevaluations of the statistical models, and paying more attention to cluster analyses) and labeled as follows: precontemplation, contemplation, preparation, action, and maintenance.[28] Relapse, which had previously been conceptualized as one of the stages is certainly a common occurrence; but rather than being understood as one of the stages of change, it is now viewed (as supported by research) as a "slide backwards" to restart the cycle at one of the earlier stages.[29]

Because Zach, as described at the beginning of the chapter, is at the first stage (precontemplation) with regard to his smoking behavior, he provides a good model for illustrating each of the stages in the Transtheoretical Model of Change. As we meet him, he is not considering or contemplating change. He is minimally aware of his health risks (the possibility of developing lung cancer and/or heart disease from smoking) but doesn't view them as particularly important. If Zach became more aware of how serious his health risks actually are (perhaps if a close friend who also smokes is diagnosed with lung cancer), he would move into the contemplation stage. In the contemplation stage, Zach would be more fully aware of the issues that confront him and may start thinking about, or contemplating, various strategies that he could use to ameliorate his risks. In the third stage, preparation, Zach would solidify a plan for action and, perhaps, seek advice or other help from family, peers,

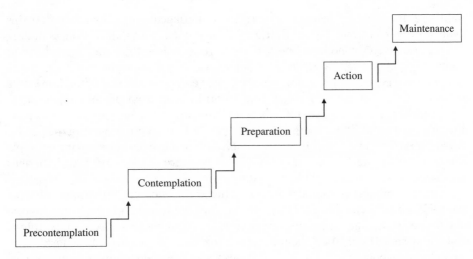

Figure 1.4 Transtheoretical model of change.

or members of a healthcare team. Zach's plans might involve using a nicotine patch or gum, asking friends and family to encourage and support him, taking on new activities to distract him from his desire to smoke, and avoiding places where other people are smoking. Then, during the fourth stage (action), Zach would begin to actually carry out his plan. During the last stage, called maintenance, Zach would continue his "action" plan, avoiding pitfalls that might cause him to lapse or relapse, working to make his new behaviors truly habitual and fully integrated into his lifestyle, and modifying his plan as his life changes.

Of course, Zach's example is a simple, linear one involving a straightforward, well-defined behavior—smoking. The reality is that many behaviors are not as straightforward and well-defined as "smoking or not" but may involve varying degrees of success at avoiding cigarettes. People seldom proceed through the changes as we have described above. Instead, people typically *cycle* through the stages, showing progress and then regression, and having less clearly defined indicators of success or failure. The individual's goal is to exhibit a general trend toward greater success over time,[28] such as by cutting back on the number of cigarettes per day and maintaining the lower level. One of the health professional's most vital roles is encouraging this progress.

Much of the research literature on the stages-of-change model addresses addictive behaviors like smoking, as in our above example with Zach. It is not entirely clear that all of the lower-order constructs (e.g., consciousness-raising, reinforcement management) have the same meaning when other types of behavior change are the focus. For example, in a meta-analysis applying the Transtheoretical Model of Change in 71 published studies on physical activity, researchers attempted to differentiate between processes of change that were experiential (consciousness-raising) and those that were behavioral (reinforcement management). They found that this distinction was not meaningful in the exercise domain and that in understanding exercise, the stage-by-process interactions were less clear than they have been in studies of psychotherapy and addictive behavior.[30]

For some primary prevention behaviors like exercise, the most "busy" or active behavior change steps occurred during the transition from precontemplation to contemplation, suggesting that the most difficult part of changing exercise behavior (or making other lifestyle changes aimed at prevention) might be getting the person to even consider increasing physical activity. This differs from our smoking example where the risks and benefits of quitting may be more obvious but the challenges associated with planning and implementation may be greater.

The Transtheoretical Model serves to highlight two very important concepts about health behavior change. First, verbal communication and cognitive processing in the early stages of change are important. What people think, and the things that they say about their health, really do matter. Second, Prochaska and DiClemente hypothesized that if a clinician's focus and direction is too divergent from the client's or if the two are working at different levels of the change process, the client can become resistant to change.[26] People are particularly likely to drop out of therapy, or quit behavior change efforts, when their expectations and those of their practitioners are quite disparate. Thus, effective communication is not only an important facilitator of early-stage change, it may be *the key* to establishing the appropriate level at which client and clinician can target their common efforts.

Social Cognitive Models

The concepts of classical conditioning[31] and operant conditioning (behavior modification[32]) combine with an emphasis on cognitive processing to form the foundation for Social Cognitive Models. Sometimes labeled Social Learning Theories,[33, 34] these approaches posit that both personal expectancies and environmental factors (e.g., reinforcements) determine behavior, and that modifying *either* of these can result in behavioral change.

Expectancies may be of several kinds. Individuals might expect that certain events are related to each other *causally* (that is, in terms of cause and effect). They might have "outcome expectations" about the *consequences* of personal action. And individuals might have expectancies of the likelihood of their own personal success (the *self-efficacy* we introduced previously). In all of these cases, expectations about what is likely to "happen next" can influence attitudes, intentions, and behaviors.

Similarly, the environments in which a person lives, works, and plays provide feedback to the individual. Some behaviors are met with praise or other rewards, while other behaviors result in less positive outcomes. The outcomes associated with behaviors serve to encourage or discourage similar behaviors in the future; thus, managing behavioral consequences is one way of influencing the behaviors themselves.

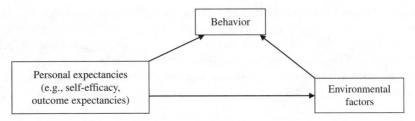

Figure 1.5 Social cognitive theory.

There are some similarities between Social Cognitive Models and the Health Belief Model.[5] As a group, Social Cognitive Models hold as crucially important the inclusion of cognitive elements such as self-efficacy (also an important component of the HBM). Other cognitive factors, including beliefs about the causes of various outcomes and the sense that things can be controlled, also warrant attention according to Social Cognitive Models.

Self-regulation (which includes things like self-reflection and observational learning) provides an additional mechanism for achieving desired outcomes and maintaining changes over time. Strategies such as learning through observation and reflecting on one's successes and failures, along with a good understanding of other cognitive processes (such as how we see causes and effects) represent a set of tools that can be quite useful when working toward health behavior change and treatment adherence. Perhaps Alex, whose health behaviors are strong, has benefited from some of these, including observational learning, his own beliefs about the links between behavior and outcome, and self-reflection.

Although people like Alex seem to easily accomplish their aims and smoothly glide through life, Alex has most likely worked hard to create what appears to be an effortless, natural, and enviable existence. Perhaps Alex's parents were good role models, showing him from an early age, through their actions, what healthy food choices and "family exercise time" were all about. Perhaps Alex still remembers one or two shockingly salient examples of uncles, aunts, or grandparents who engaged in poor health behaviors and experienced debilitating illness or death as a result. Maybe, through painful experience, Alex has learned to set manageable goals and to monitor his own progress toward achieving them. We simply don't know. What we can say is that each of these elements, and more, are important in setting the foundation upon which future behaviors will be built.

An individual's own unique experiences, beliefs, and personal attributes influence his or her responses to new information, to environmental reinforcements, to motivational messages, and to all of the other things that are potential triggers for behavioral change. In every application of theoretical models to the motivation and management of real people, close attention must be paid to personal characteristics and the ways in which these alter the meaning of environmental factors for an individual. Close attention to the "person by environment interaction" will allow behavior change strategies to be tailored to the individual, thus optimizing the likelihood of successful change. Failure to attend to this interaction may result in plans for change that do not accurately reflect the individual's views, beliefs, motivations, and expectations. Interventions such as these have a lower likelihood of success, even if they seem to be well conceived. The interplay between personal characteristics and external factors is addressed in more detail in Chapter 4.

Precaution Adoption Process Model

Like the Transtheoretical Model of Change, the Precaution Adoption Process Model is a stage model, focusing on an individual's change over time, rather than on predicting levels of behavior across individuals. It is aimed specifically at understanding reactions to health hazards and the initiation of new or more complex precautionary health behaviors. This model, formally proposed in 1988, presumes seven specific stages, some of which are similar to those described in the Transtheoretical Model of Change. In the Precaution Adoption Process Model, the individual is first unaware, then aware but disengaged, then engaged and deciding what action to take, then deciding to act (or not to act, at least not yet), then acting, and finally maintaining the adopted behavior.[35, 36] Just as optimal strategies are proposed to vary by stage, barriers to change have also been found, in several studies, to differ according to stage.[36–38]

For example, in 1992 Neil Weinstein[36] applied this theory to the issue of lung cancer risks associated with naturally occurring radon gas and precautions that might be taken to reduce radon gas exposure in the home. He suggested that in the first stages of this model a person is not aware of radon gas and its associated risks. Once radon gas is learned about, the individual's initial reaction may depend upon his or her sense that it is personally relevant. The next stages involve the individual recognizing that he or she is indeed at risk, followed by identifying precautionary steps that might be taken (such as increasing ventilation in the home to reduce radon exposure), and finally, following through and implementing those precautionary measures.

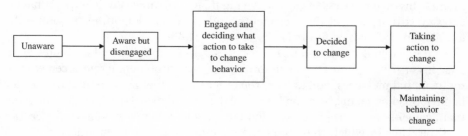

Figure 1.6 Precaution adoption process model.

and apply systematic behavior change methods that are supported by research evidence. An unsystematic, unproven approach may not be effective.

Ideally, theories should be used in ways that complement each other. For instance, it is as important to understand people's beliefs about their own risks as it is to understand where they are in terms of their "readiness" to change. It is also important to tailor interventions to the type of behaviors that are being targeted. For example, the challenges associated with the primary preventive behavior of wearing sunscreen (to reduce the risk of skin cancer) are different from the challenges of adherence to a rigorous and unpleasant chemotherapy regimen for malignant melanoma. Throughout this book we will detail the specific elements of the information-motivation-strategy model. We will discuss "informing" as it relates to providing information so that it can be understood and remembered (especially in Chapter 3), evaluating information about health risks and outcomes (the major focus of Chapter 5), and using technology as an aid (in Chapter 7). We will focus on better understanding the concept of "motivating," specifically as it involves persuading someone to adopt a goal and encouraging its pursuit (primarily in Chapter 2). And, we will evaluate many different methods for effectively "strategizing," both in terms of specific methods for developing good habits (Chapter 4) and in terms of techniques that health-care providers can use to help people change (especially in Chapters 6 and 8).

References

1. Elias WS, Murphy RJ. The case for health promotion programs containing health care costs: a review of the literature. Am J Occup Ther. 1986 Nov;40(11):759–63.
2. Ajzen I, Fishbein M. Understanding Attitudes and Predicting Social Behavior. Englewood Cliffs, NJ: Prentice Hall; 1980.
3. Rosenstock IM. Historical origins of the Health Belief Model. Health Education Monographs. 1974;2(4).
4. Becker MH, Maiman LA. Sociobehavioral determinants of compliance with health and medical care recommendations. Med Care. 1975 Jan;13(1):10–24.
5. Rosenstock IM, Strecher VJ, Becker MH. Social learning theory and the Health Belief Model. Health Educ Q. 1988 Summer;15(2):175–83.
6. Janz NK, Becker MH. The Health Belief Model: a decade later. Health Educ Behav. 1984 January 1, 1984;11(1):1–47.
7. Wallace LS. Osteoporosis prevention in college women: application of the expanded Health Belief Model. Am J Health Behav. 2002 May–Jun;26(3):163–72.
8. Aljasem LI, Peyrot M, Wissow L, Rubin RR. The impact of barriers and self-efficacy on self-care behaviors in type 2 diabetes. Diabetes Educ. 2001 May–Jun;27(3):393–404.
9. DiMatteo MR, Haskard KB, Williams SL. Health beliefs, disease severity, and patient adherence: a meta-analysis. Med Care. 2007 Jun;45(6):521–8.
10. Fishbein M, Ajzen, I. Belief, Attitude, Intention, and Behavior: An Introduction to Theory and Research. Reading, MA: Addison-Wesley; 1975.

11. Sheppard BH, Hartwick, J, Warshaw, PL. The theory of reasoned action: A meta-analysis of past research with recommendations of modifications and future research. J Consum Res. 1988;15:325–43.
12. Albarracin D, Johnson BT, Fishbein M, Muellerleile PA. Theories of Reasoned Action and Planned Behavior as models of condom use: a meta-analysis. Psychol Bull. 2001 Jan;127(1):142–61.
13. Hagger MS, Chatzisarantis NL, Biddle SJ. The influence of autonomous and controlling motives on physical activity intentions within the Theory of Planned Behaviour. Br J Health Psychol. 2002 Sep;7(Part 3):283–97.
14. Doll J, Orth B. The Fishbein and Ajzen Theory of Reasoned Action applied to contraceptive behavior: model variants and meaningfulness. J Appl Soc Psychol. 1993;23(5):395–415.
15. Fisher WA, Fisher JD, Rye BJ. Understanding and promoting AIDS-preventive behavior: insights from the Theory of Reasoned Action. Health Psychol. 1995 May;14(3):255–64.
16. Godin G, Kok G. The Theory of Planned Behavior: a review of its applications to health-related behaviors. Am J Health Promot. 1996 Nov–Dec;11(2):87–98.
17. Hillhouse JJ, Stair AW, 3rd, Adler CM. Predictors of sunbathing and sunscreen use in college undergraduates. J Behav Med. 1996 Dec;19(6):543–61.
18. Montano DE, Taplin SH. A test of an expanded Theory of Reasoned Action to predict mammography participation. Soc Sci Med. 1991;32(6):733–41.
19. Ajzen I. From intentions to actions: a Theory of Planned Behavior. In: Beckman JKJ, editor. Action-control: From Cognition to Behavior. Heidelberg: Springer; 1985. p. 11–39.
20. Ajzen I. The Theory of Planned Behavior. Organizational Behavior and Human Decision Processes 1991;50:179–211.
21. Hausenblas HA, Carron AV, Mack DE. Application of the Theories of Reasoned Action and Planned Behavior to exercise behavior: A meta-analysis. J Sport Exercise Psychol. 1997;19(1):36–51.
22. Madden TJ, Ellen PS, Ajzen I. A comparison of the Theory of Planned Behavior and the Theory of Reasoned Action. Pers Soc Psychol Bull. 1992;18(1):3–9.
23. Armitage CJ, Conner M. Efficacy of the Theory of Planned Behaviour: a meta-analytic review. Br J Soc Psychol. 2001 Dec;40(Pt 4):471–99.
24. Terry DJ, Hogg MA. Group norms and the attitude-behavior relationship: a role for group identification. Pers Soc Psychol Bull. 1996 August 1;22(8):776–93.
25. Prochaska J. Systems of Psychotherapy: A Transtheoretical Analysis. Homewood, IL: Dorsey Press; 1979.
26. Prochaska JO, DiClemente CC. Transtheoretical therapy: Toward a more integrative model of change. Psychotherapy: Theory, Research and Practice. 1982;19(3):276–88.
27. Prochaska JO, DiClemente CC. Stages and processes of self-change of smoking: toward an integrative model of change. J Consult Clin Psychol. 1983 Jun;51(3):390–5.
28. Prochaska JO, DiClemente CC, Norcross JC. In search of how people change. Applications to addictive behaviors. Am Psychol. 1992 Sep;47(9):1102–14.
29. DiClemente CC, Prochaska JO, Fairhurst SK, Velicer WF, Velasquez MM, Rossi JS. The process of smoking cessation: an analysis of precontemplation, contemplation, and preparation stages of change. J Consult Clin Psychol. 1991 Apr;59(2):295–304.
30. Marshall SJ, Biddle SJ. The Transtheoretical Model of behavior change: a meta-analysis of applications to physical activity and exercise. Ann Behav Med. 2001 Fall;23(4):229–46.

31. Pavlov I. Conditioned Reflexes: An Investigation of the Physiological Activity of the Cerebral Cortex. London: Oxford University Press; 1927.
32. Bandura A. Principles of Behavior Modification. New York: Holt, Rinehart, & Winston; 1969.
33. Bandura A. Social Learning Theory. Englewood Cliffs, NJ: Prentice Hall; 1977.
34. Rotter JB. Social Learning and Clinical Psychology. New York: Prentice Hall; 1954.
35. Weinstein ND. The Precaution Adoption Process. Health Psychol. 1988;7(4):355–86.
36. Weinstein ND, Sandman PM. A model of the Precaution Adoption Process: evidence from home radon testing. Health Psychol. 1992;11(3):170–80.
37. Blalock SJ, DeVellis RF, Giorgino KB, DeVellis BM, Gold DT, Dooley MA, Anderson JJ, Smith SL. Osteoporosis prevention in premenopausal women: using a stage model approach to examine the predictors of behavior. Health Psychol. 1996 Mar;15(2):84–93.
38. Weinstein ND, Lyon JE, Sandman PM, Cuite CL. Experimental evidence for stages of health behavior change: the precaution adoption process model applied to home radon testing. Health Psychol. 1998 Sep;17(5):445–53.
39. DiMatteo MR, DiNicola DD. Achieving Patient Compliance. New York: Pergamon Press; 1982.

2

Persuading and Motivating Positive Health Behaviors

How soon "not now" becomes "never."
—Martin Luther, Protestant Reformer

Goal Setting

In Chapter 1 we outlined several important theoretical models that underpin our knowledge of behavioral change toward the goal of health. These models lead us to some practical questions about what factors persuade an individual to adopt particular health-related goals and what factors keep the individual motivated to pursue these goals.

Sometimes people target certain health objectives because of their emotions and feelings; other times they are driven by social comparisons, logical reasoning, or even some kind of direct pressure. An individual might suddenly *feel* compelled to undertake a challenge, such as training to run a 10-kilometer (k) race, after spending the afternoon watching the track and field events of the summer Olympics. Inspiration from watching the athletes may propel the individual to plan a workout schedule to achieve the level of cardiovascular fitness and stamina that a 10k race would require. Sometimes, though, people adopt goals that are rooted in social comparisons, such as when a parent observes other parents swimming with their children and then decides to join in for both exercise and fun.

Sometimes health goals are undertaken after a well-reasoned decision-making process has been completed, such as when one decides to change several behaviors at the same time to achieve greater cardiovascular health. The available information and data are likely to support the goal, and clearly seem to outweigh any arguments against their adoption. Take the example of Gene. He has recently been diagnosed with worryingly high LDL ("bad") cholesterol and hypertension. Together these conditions place him at high risk for cardiovascular disease. He needs to make some sweeping dietary changes and increase his level of daily exercise. In addition, his physician has recommended that he begin taking two medications that will help lower his cholesterol and control his high blood pressure. Gene has accepted this advice and has set several health-related goals for himself. He has the long-term goals of lowering blood pressure and cholesterol, and the short-term goals of consistently taking his medications, walking each evening after work, and replacing some of the fattening foods in his diet with more fresh fruits and vegetables. Gene believes that each of these goals is achievable, despite the possibility of unpleasant side effects associated with one of his prescribed medications. In weighing the potential risks and benefits, Gene judges the arguments in favor of taking medication to be stronger than the arguments against it.

Often, health goals are adopted in response to some form of persuasion. It is common for people to be influenced by media campaigns or by popular press articles that report research findings from scientific articles. For example, a journalist might write about the copious research evidence supporting sleep as crucial for health and longevity. Eric Nagourney, for example, has presented compelling evidence in the *New York Times* that disrupted sleep patterns are associated with problems regulating blood sugar and might be linked to diabetes. He cites empirical data published in the *Proceedings of the National Academy of Sciences*,[1] and presents evidence that is compelling enough to motivate an individual to change behavior and pursue the goal of healthy sleep. Many of our own students, after reading the *New York Times* article, were convinced of the importance of sleep and said that they would make a concerted effort to get enough of it! Of course, we've also talked with students who are committed to other, somewhat more dubious behavior changes as a result of compelling news articles or television exposés. These include using herbal supplements that claim to be "fat-busters," and adhering to methods of exercise that are supposed to make a person look like an Olympic athlete in only five minutes a day!

Having adequate health information available to make good decisions and to set reasonable health goals is important; the availability of good health information helps people to be more "health literate."[2] Studies show that accurate information about the risks and benefits of particular health behaviors actually does influence people's choices about their own behaviors. We discuss this issue in more detail later in this chapter and in Chapter 5, where we consider how individuals weigh information about the risks and benefits of health action. Here, we note that having good health information is essential, although it is only part of the equation; many people fail to set or effectively pursue good health-related goals despite their knowledge.[3] Information is the crucial *first step* because people need to *know what to do* in order to make changes in the right direction.

Goals are formed and driven by a combination of reason and emotion. Yet sometimes even convincing evidence *and* a strong emotional appeal are not enough. A person likely also needs to feel confident that it is *possible* for him or her to achieve the identified goal. We encountered this concept, referred to as *self-efficacy*, in Chapter 1, and it plays a central role in determining both the goals that people set for themselves and the actions they are willing to take to achieve those goals.

In the first part of this chapter, then, we examine the complexity of knowledge, emotion, and confidence, among other factors that contribute to making a goal worth pursuing. We consider the factors that compel us to embrace some challenges and to avoid others. Later in the chapter, we discuss what motivates people to *take action* in pursuit of a worthy health goal once that goal has been adopted.

Social Comparisons

Since psychologist Leon Festinger first described his theory of social comparison processes in 1954, researchers have been interested in how various kinds of social comparisons influence people's emotions and behaviors.[4] Every person engages in social comparisons; and the effects those comparisons have on health (and other outcomes) can be positive or negative depending on the circumstances. Researchers have paid particular attention to how different aspects of emotion, goal-setting, and motivation are associated with upward and downward comparisons. *Upward comparisons* are those in which a person compares him- or herself with someone else (either real or hypothetical) who is "better off" than they are on a particular dimension or set of dimensions. For example, one might compare oneself with someone who is more accomplished at a particular sport, is more physically fit, or is more successful at sticking to a healthy eating plan. Alternatively, *downward comparisons* are those in which the person looks to a reference group or person who is "worse off" than they are. For example, one might compare oneself to those who never exercise, are quite obese, or are more severely ill with the same disease.

Downward comparisons have sometimes been linked to more positive emotional states[5–7] because they tend to make us feel better about ourselves. Our own difficulties can be put into perspective and the things we are thankful for can be highlighted. But downward comparisons tend not to serve as potent motivators because they focus attention on obstacles or goals that have already been surmounted or achieved.[8,9] Downward comparisons can cause us to become complacent about our own health behaviors. We might be doing better than some other people, but still not doing very well!

In providing a picture of what "could be," upward comparisons, in contrast, can energize a person to action.[8,9] But they can also foster a sense of discouragement if there is a wide gap between one's current state and the comparison point. This is especially likely if an individual does not recognize their own personal progress toward the higher level that others seem to have already achieved.[10,11]

We cannot accurately predict how any one individual will react to upward and downward comparisons in his or her own health behaviors. Other factors such as a person's self-esteem and perceived control over situations can further complicate individual emotional reactions to comparisons with how other people are doing.[5] Most studies, though, do find that upward comparisons inspire the setting of more ambitious[9] goals and that downward comparisons are able to ameliorate negative moods for those with low self-esteem.[12]

Let's consider an example. Ardis has low self-esteem and is feeling overwhelmed by all of the changes she needs to make in order to get her weight under control. She is 70 pounds overweight, and knows that she needs to both change her diet and start exercising. But her knees hurt when she tries to "power-walk," and she easily gets a side-ache and becomes short-of-breath. These obstacles to exercise seem almost insurmountable and leave her feeling badly about herself.

At a recent meeting of her newly joined exercise support group, Ardis met several people who are in worse shape than she is. Three of them are actually categorized as "morbidly obese" which corresponds to a body mass index (BMI) of 40 or above. These individuals are approximately 100 pounds above their ideal body weight. During the group session, Ardis listened to them talk about their own difficulties with exercise and she began to feel that there was hope for her. After all, her situation was not as extreme as theirs. Her downward comparison improved her helpless mood and gave her a sense that exercise was something that she could indeed do if she persisted or took it a day at a time. Fortunately, she did not become complacent about her own health just because she was not as overweight as others.

The role of upward and downward comparisons can be even further complicated by the individual's perceived control. Research shows that comparisons, either upward or downward, are less likely to induce positive mood states for those who perceive that they have little control over their own outcomes.[5,8,13] The likely results of upward and downward comparisons in the presence of different levels of perceived control are illustrated in Figure 2.1. If Ardis, during her group meeting, believed that she couldn't exert any control over her exercise regimen and instead felt that she, herself, was on a track toward morbid obesity, she would have been much less likely to experience an improvement in her mood. Instead of being uplifting, the recognition of her situation as less dire than others might have been discouraging; she may have seen only her own imagined future in her morbidly obese peers.

Another member of Ardis' group, Pat, is also about 70 pounds overweight, but she makes an upward comparison, focusing on a group member who, after a year in the program, is now only 20 pounds away from her ideal weight. Pat feels that she does have control over her outcomes, and she is motivated to achieve a similar goal. The upward comparison is a very invigorating and motivating experience for her. If Pat had low perceived control over her own weight-related outcomes, however, this upward comparison would likely have been overwhelming and disheartening rather than inspiring.

Research on social comparison underscores for us the fact that a person's characteristics must be well understood before specific types of comparisons can be encouraged to prompt the adoption of health-related goals. We must first ask the question, does this person currently have high self-esteem? Does the individual perceive that they have control over their behaviors? Do they see the comparison person or group as similar to themselves? Are they optimistic? Easily discouraged?

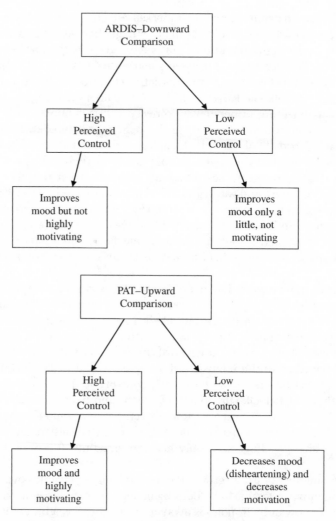

Figure 2.1 Upward and downward comparisons in the presence of low or high perceived behavioral control.

Intrinsically motivated? The answers to these questions are essential if healthcare professionals are to encourage comparisons that will be most helpful to a specific person. Suggesting that someone strive to achieve what another has accomplished may or may not be helpful, depending upon many factors. For example, the relevance and influence of social comparisons depends to some degree on the perceived similarity of others. Comparisons with those who seem very different are less useful because there is little reason to believe that one's own trajectory or outcome would be similar, regardless of behavior. Thus, social comparisons operate against the backdrop of an individual's already-present tendencies, perceptions, strengths, and weaknesses and within the context of the person's life. Social comparisons do not operate in a vacuum.

Social comparisons are also not "still snapshots." People usually receive feedback over time about where they stand relative to others as they work to achieve their various goals. There are two categories of basic possibilities for what are called "self-other performance patterns" and their associated comparisons. These categories are "static" and "dynamic." In the static comparison category, an individual could consistently perform in one of three ways compared with peers: *(1)* better than, *(2)* worse than, or *(3)* the same as peers. In the dynamic comparison category, an individual could experience *(1)* progressive decline in performance relative to peers; or a person could demonstrate *(2)* growing mastery as compared to peers. The feedback that one receives about her or his performance relative to others (e.g., what one is told by one's doctor about health markers or how one "measures up" during monthly weigh-ins at a weight-loss group) is important. Such feedback contributes to subsequent goal-setting and self-efficacy. For example, someone might be told they are quite physically fit for their age, or conversely that most people their age are getting more exercise than they are. Not surprisingly, feedback indicating that one is improving seems to have an empowering effect and tends to be associated with higher self-efficacy and clearer thinking, and with setting higher subsequent goals. On the other hand, feedback that suggests one is losing ground or not meeting expectations can accelerate a downward spiral because it lowers the individual's sense of self-efficacy and leads to deteriorating performance.[14]

This concept is illustrated in Table 2.1 with Ardis, Pat, and another member of their group. Although Ardis's performance is initially at the same level as the rest of the group (matching the average), over time her trend is toward less weight loss. Even though she is still losing weight, she is not losing as much as her peers over time. This is likely to undermine her sense of self-efficacy and to result in continued underperformance and a tendency to set less ambitious goals in the future. Pat's experience is the opposite. Her first weigh-in also places her right at the group average, but she demonstrates a consistent pattern of achievement that fosters her sense of self-efficacy, encourages her to set higher goals in the future, and increases her chances of future successes. Emory's case is perhaps the most illustrative of the importance of feedback regarding improvement. His weight loss is consistently below the group average, yet his performance pattern demonstrates regular progress at each weigh-in. This is likely to increase his self-efficacy as well as his future goal-setting and performance even though he never outperforms the group, although these effects will probably not be as dramatic as they are for Pat.

So, what can be done to help Ardis? Does her downward performance pattern doom her to ultimate failure? Not necessarily! An astute group leader might take a little extra time with Ardis to help redirect her comparisons. Instead of pointing out how Ardis is doing relative to her group's average, she might instead compare her

Table 2.1 Self-other performance patterns for weight loss and associated outcomes.

Patient	February	March	April	Self-efficacy	Performance	Goal-setting
Ardis	Weight loss is equal to the group average	Loses 2 pounds less than group average	Loses 3.5 pounds less than group average	Decreasing over time	Decreasing over time	Likely to be less ambitious
Pat	Weight loss is equal to the group average	Weight loss 1.5 pounds more than group average	Weight loss 2 pounds more than group average	Increasing over time	Maintaining or increasing over time	Likely to be more ambitious
Emory	Loses 4 pounds less than group average	Loses 2 pounds less than group average	Weight loss is nearly equal to group average	Increasing over time	Maintaining or increasing	Likely to be more ambitious

performance to that of another group, such as those in the general public (who are not part of a weight-loss group). Or, the group leader might point out that it's common to experience a plateau in weight loss, or that Ardis's weight loss has slowed but has *not* reached a plateau. This strategy will help increase Ardis' self-efficacy and may help put her back on a more successful trajectory, or at least deflect discouragement and help her maintain her current level of performance. Thus, in addition to social comparisons, feedback can be managed to optimize success, including redirecting toward more constructive comparisons.

Persuasive Messages

Social psychology has provided us with a great deal of evidence about what types of messages are most likely to be persuasive (you will find these summarized in Table 2.2). You will probably not be surprised to hear that the message is not the only element that is important. The messenger who tries to persuade is also crucial. There are two primary characteristics that make a messenger persuasive: the individual's expertise and our liking for the person. Let us look at each of these in a bit more detail.

Table 2.2 Summary of elements of persuasive messages.

Messenger Expertise	This is the perception that the messenger has special knowledge and experience and that therefore their message is worth paying attention to. It can be indicated by many things such as a degree or title, professional clothing, and so on. Expert status can be effectively used by health-care professionals of all types.
Liking for the Messenger	People who are liked are better able to persuade others; attractive individuals, those who are seen as being similar to self, and those who are familiar tend to be best liked. Making the effort to build familiarity and trust, and to point out parallels between the professional and the patient can serve to make the health-care professional's message more persuasive.
Perceptions of Scarcity	When opportunities to gain or obtain something are limited, they are often more highly valued than those that are commonly and easily available. Emphasizing the need to act quickly may motivate patients away from procrastination.
Norm of Reciprocity	It is natural to feel the need to reciprocate, whether that means returning a compliment or repaying a good deed. This tendency can be used to encourage a variety of good health behaviors in patients.
Desire to be Consistent	People generally like to maintain consistency between their beliefs and actions, and across behaviors. Getting patients to make a commitment or to initiate a positive pattern (even if the first step is quite small) can be a powerful motivator of future health behaviors.
Fear Induction	Introducing anxiety or fear regarding the negative outcomes of poor health behaviors can be an effective strategy for motivating change, but only if the fear induced is not overwhelming and clear, manageable steps for avoiding the frightening outcome are provided.
Teachable Moments	People's own experiences and life events (or those of people they are close to) can often make the need for a change more salient. Keeping track of what is going on in a patient's personal life may create opportunities to teach and motivate more effectively.
Message Framing	Persuasive messages may be framed in terms of what may be gained if a health behavior is adopted, or what may be lost if one is not. Which type of framing is most effective will depend on the type of health behavior that is being targeted.
Expectations	People's expectations for what will happen if they perform (or don't perform) a certain behavior influence whether or not that behavior is attempted. Their perceptions about what important others in their lives will think about the behavior are also important influences on behavioral adoption.

Expertise

We know that when information is provided by someone deemed to have expertise on a topic, it carries more weight than if that same information is conveyed by someone without expertise.[15] Some individuals have authority by virtue of their knowledge and past experience and the label *expert power* is often used to describe this form of influence.[16,17] Other forms of social influence that medical experts often use are *informational power* (that based on the content of the expert's communication), *reward power* (the capacity to give rewards), *coercive power* (the capacity to withhold rewards), and *referent power* (the capacity to provide an appropriate reference point for the patient). Examples of each of these can be found in Table 2.3.

That these various forms of power are effective is good news for those in health care; physicians, nurses, dentists, pharmacists, and so many other health professionals who encourage health behavior change already have the appropriate expertise, information, reward resources, and anecdotal examples to be convincing. They are in a perfect position to help persuade their patients to pursue good health behaviors! [18]

Table 2.3 Examples of persuasive power in use.

Expert Power	"In my experience, Katrina, people with blood pressure levels as high as yours usually can't control their hypertension with diet and exercise alone. I've seen a lot of cases like this and, trust me, medication really will help."
Informational Power	"Mona, despite the fact that you feel healthy, your fasting plasma glucose results are back and show that you're again above the cutoff of 126 mg per dL. I also see, in examining your retinas that there seem to be small changes occurring. The damage isn't severe enough to qualify as diabetic retinopathy yet, but regulating your blood glucose is now more crucial than ever."
Reward Power	"We've got a new incentive program for those in our 'walk fit' group, Curtis. Those who walk an extra 5,000 steps per week over the next month will get two free tickets to the County Health Expo! Do you want to sign on for that?"
Coercive Power	"I'm sorry Mr. Balcom, but I can't make that referral for you until we can get your weight within the target range. I know that you're in a lot of pain but it simply makes no sense to undergo knee replacement surgery when you're this heavy."
Referent Power	"Victor, I struggle to eat right, too—believe me, I enjoy burgers and fries as much as the next person. But I made a commitment to follow this eating plan almost ten years ago now. It took me nearly a year of small steps and changes to get it right, but I'm now at the point where I can resist the temptation to snack between meals and I honestly feel that I enjoy my occasional 'splurges' more than I used to, because I don't have a guilty conscience about them."

Liking

Many studies also demonstrate that when a messenger is well liked, their persuasive power is greater.[15] We tend to like people who we think are attractive,[19] whom we perceive as similar to us,[20] and with whom we are more familiar.[21] Although attractiveness may not be easily changeable, the latter two characteristics are easier to target. Health-care providers may be able to increase their perceptions of similarity and familiarity by briefly sharing some of their own experiences with their patients (e.g., by pointing out their own challenges in increasing their exercise). The mere fact of creating a "therapeutic alliance" over time will increase familiarity and the sense of comfort within the mutual interaction. Thus, each member of the healthcare team should be encouraged to work to establish trusting, supportive relationships with their patients.

Scarcity, Reciprocity, and Consistency

In addition to coming from a well-liked expert, the most persuasive messages tend to involve some of the following: *(1)* perceptions of scarcity (such as, when someone believes that an opportunity is "now or never"); *(2)* norms of reciprocity (the desire to return in kind what one receives); and *(3)* the desire to be consistent in one's behaviors. Each of these principles can be used in formulating and delivering persuasive messages to patients, thus helping them to set and commit to health-related goals.

For example, suppose that a nurse educator believes his patient would benefit from a 2-hour seminar on the self-management of diabetes. He might encourage the patient to make the commitment to attend by pointing out, truthfully of course, that there are only a few open spaces left for the upcoming session and that it will be several weeks before another session will be scheduled. The fact that only a few vacancies remain, and that quick action is required to secure one of them, may make them seem more appealing to the patient.

One illustration of the norm of reciprocity is a token gift from the medical office. A physician might, for example, provide her patients with a refrigerator magnet that serves as a picture frame and has a "dry erase" area where the next appointment can be written in. This small gift is likely to be appreciated, and the patient may feel obliged to return the kindness by keeping appointments, or calling early if an appointment needs to be rescheduled. Or, perhaps this same physician, when making a referral, might emphasize the fact that she is referring to a very talented specialist and highlight past experience with this individual; the patient may feel particularly grateful and inclined to reciprocate by promptly making and keeping an appointment.

Finally, particular behaviors can be highlighted by the health-care provider to encourage consistency in healthy behavior patterns. For example, a nutritionist might reiterate the ways in which the patient has already decreased the sodium in her diet and remind the patient of her own statements about wanting to cut down on salt. This serves as a way of illustrating how reasonable the next dietary steps might be, and reinforcing the fact that the patient is able to demonstrate consistency and perseverance.

The human desire to remain consistent and keep commitments can also be used once the treatment plan has been devised by encouraging the patient to participate in the creation of a *behavioral contract.* A behavioral contract outlines the plan that the patient is committing to follow, and it is then signed by both parties, indicating the importance placed on the behavior by both the health-care professional and the patient. The patient's desire to maintain consistency with what has previously been agreed to may create subtle pressure to adhere, as well as to adopt other health behaviors later on that are consistent with the aims of the signed contract.

Fear Induction

Another important, but often misused, persuasive technique is fear induction. Fear messages are complex, and although they are potentially powerful motivators, using fear-inducing tactics can also backfire. A meta-analysis of the literature on "fear appeals" (i.e., messages that are specifically meant to induce fear in the recipient) shows that fear-provoking messages are the most emotionally powerful of all types of messages, but that in order to be effective they must be paired with equally powerful information about how one might circumvent the feared outcome.[22] People must not only be provided with information about how to avoid what they fear, but this information must also be framed in a way that maximizes the individual's sense of self-efficacy. That is, the individual must be confident that he or she is *able* to minimize the threat.

When people are simply frightened, they are not likely to engage in preventive health behaviors. Instead, their fear activates defensive responses such as avoidance or reactance.[22] A strong body of research on this topic suggests that trying to simply scare a person into health behavior change (e.g., telling them they will die if they keep smoking and showing them graphic photos of horrible cancers and emaciated sufferers) is unlikely to be successful without the provision of a clear set of steps to take in order to stop smoking and achieve better health.

Teachable Moments

As with so many things in life, timing is important, and there are times in life when people are particularly receptive to making changes to improve their health. These are called "teachable moments" and they tend to have two things in common: *(1)* an emotionally motivating component, such as a "close call" or a friend's diabetes diagnosis; and *(2)* a reasoned realization that change is necessary, such as when the emotionally charged event leads to a closer examination of one's own risks and the possible ways in which one might minimize those risks.[23] For example, a person may be motivated to eat a healthier diet and exercise regularly after finding out that his best friend was diagnosed with diabetes.

care for your family") can be an effective way of prompting efforts toward a health-related goal. Even something as simple as mentioning the name of someone (e.g., mother, father, or a close friend) who has an interest in a particular goal has been shown to influence people's commitment to that goal.[29] This effect is most powerful when the relationship is close between the two people, but care must be taken not to associate too many goals with any single person. Too many associations can dilute that person's power to motivate goal commitment.

Case Study Box 2.1—Analysis of How Gene's Subjective Norms and Other Health Beliefs Influence His Goal Adoption

Gene has high blood pressure and high LDL cholesterol. His medical recommendations include dietary changes, more regular exercise, and medication.

Social Context	Norm or Evaluation	Value to Gene
Gene's daughter	Supports change	High
Gene's wife	Supports change	High
Gene's best friend	Neutral	High
Gene's coworkers	Neutral	Moderate
Gene's physician	Supports change	High

Health Belief	Salience to Gene	Value to Gene
High LDLs and blood pressure place me at significant health risk	High	High
Eating more fresh fruits and vegetables will be expensive	High	High
My medications are expensive	High	High
Taking prescribed medications will reduce my risk for disease	High	High
Side effects of my medications will make my coworkers avoid me	Moderate	Low
Reducing the fat in my diet will improve my health	Low	Moderate
I am capable of making the changes necessary to improve my health	High	High

In terms of his social networks, Gene is in a strong position. The most important people in his life support his desire to change and there is nobody who is actively unsupportive. It would be even better if Gene's best friend was also supportive, but the overall system of support that Gene enjoys bodes well for his success.

With regard to his health beliefs it can be seen that his expectations are generally appropriate (e.g., that certain of his current behaviors place him at risk and that making

> **Continued**
>
> changes will decrease his risk for disease) and his self-efficacy is high. The increased cost of his medications and the healthier foods he plans to eat concerns him, as does the possible embarrassment at work that the side effects (bloating, gas, and occasional diarrhea) of one of his medications might cause him. He is currently paying more attention to things that should be added to his diet (such as fresh produce) rather than thinking much about the fat content of other things he eats regularly.
>
> In all, Gene has a high likelihood of success. A health educator might work with Gene to reinforce the importance of cutting fat intake as well as increasing fresh vegetable and fruit consumption. Choosing generic medications, if available, might ease his monetary concerns or perhaps there is a program at the clinic that could help him afford the medications he needs. Taking into account his concerns about possible side effects, and being open to varying the medication regimen if necessary, can also promote Gene's success.

Goal Pursuit

Once a goal has been chosen, what motivates someone to pursue that goal despite obstacles and failures, and beyond initial successes? Several of the things that prompt initial investment in the goal also predict ongoing motivation and goal pursuit: the desires of others, the expectations of outcome success, and an individual's self-efficacy. Those who set their health goals partly on the basis of what they think others (e.g., parents, spouses, or friends) expect of them are likely to be motivated to continue pursuing their goals because of these same expectations. It is important to keep in mind, though, that not everyone is equally motivated by the expectations of others; some people really don't care much about any opinions but their own. Further, different people derive different degrees of satisfaction from goal attainment, and different degrees of distress or negative emotion when they experience failure.[30-32]

what works best for you?

Beliefs about Outcomes

What people believe about the likely outcomes of their behavior can also play an important role in determining whether they continue to persevere over time with their newly minted habits. Their optimism and their sense of self-efficacy are particularly important in their maintenance of health behaviors.

Optimism

Some people are optimistic, that is, they have a general tendency to expect positive outcomes.[33,34] Optimism, which is a traitlike characteristic, appears to be a major determinant of goal-directed behavior and tenacity. Optimistic people persevere and keep trying despite difficulties![33]

Optimism functions, however, in some apparently contradictory ways. Individuals who are optimistic expect positive outcomes, although sometimes they do not recognize the need to modify their own behaviors. In other words, optimists predict good health outcomes for themselves, even when they do little or nothing to positively change their health behaviors (An optimist might think: "This super-sized banana split is a good choice for meeting my daily fruit needs!"). Optimists can feel so good about everything that they have little motivation to change and adopt healthy behaviors. It is also the case, though, that those with optimistic self-beliefs actually see themselves as competent to make changes in their own behaviors once they decide to make those changes. Optimists feel good about their abilities, and they are more likely than nonoptimists to attempt behavioral modifications.[35]

It is also evident that optimistic self-beliefs do not operate equally across all types and phases of behavior change. Some individuals may feel quite optimistic about initiating change in some areas but not in others, or competent to start a new behavior but frustrated and pessimistic when facing the inevitable difficulties and barriers in its long-term maintenance. Others may feel that they are quite able to get back on the right track after a setback but feel less positive about their abilities in the early stages of behavior change, when they need to start something new. It is also likely that people's optimistic beliefs may be inconsistent across different types of health-relevant behaviors. Optimism may help when meeting primary prevention goals such as eating a healthful diet or when initially faced with a health crisis. Optimism may be less helpful when dealing with the ongoing challenges of treatment for a chronic illness or when making assessments about risks (such as assuming a sexual partner is disease-free and deciding not to use a condom).[34–37]

The coping strategy called *constructive thinking* has emerged as a more adaptive "cousin" to optimism, capturing much of what seems useful about optimism, while avoiding the naïve aspects of that construct. Constructive thinking involves the ability to revise thinking and solve problems (delaying gratification as necessary) under stressful situations, and to maintain a positive outlook.[38,39] The problem-solving aspects seem especially useful in predicting a range of health behaviors from substance use to behavioral adjustments during pregnancy[40,41] and improving it may foster adaptive behaviors such as adherence.[42]

Self-Efficacy

Optimistic self-beliefs are similar in many ways to self-efficacy which, as we described earlier, involves the sense that one is capable of performing the behaviors necessary to achieve a particular outcome.[43] Psychologist Albert Bandura proposed four specific sources for an individual's self-efficacy (in order of effectiveness): *(1)* past experience in performing specific behaviors (e.g., recognizing that one has been able to achieve past similar goals); *(2)* vicarious experiences (e.g., watching others who are similar to oneself successfully perform behaviors); *(3)* verbal persuasion (e.g., being told that one is capable); and *(4)* the experience of physiological arousal (e.g., an adrenaline surge conveying excitement, or conversely a racing heart suggesting fear). A high sense of self-efficacy makes it more likely that an individual will initiate a behavior, and self-efficacy, in turn, influences the degree of effort that is expended and sustained over time. Sustained effort is likely to lead to higher levels of achievement, which then further increase self-efficacy for a given task or behavior.[43] A cycle of success is thus created!

A rich body of literature shows that self-efficacy leads to better health behaviors including commitment to exercise, weight management, contraception, and decreased cigarette and alcohol use.[44] Studies also show that it is possible to change a person's sense of self-efficacy (at least over the short term) so as to enhance positive behavioral outcomes;[44-46] some techniques for doing this are summarized in Table 2.4. But keep in mind that the easiest and most frequently used method for increasing self-efficacy (verbal persuasion) is also one of the least effective. So, while it is certainly acceptable for physical therapists, nurses, or internists to verbally encourage patients, it is even more effective when they help patients to identify role models (people just like them who are facing challenges and succeeding) or when they support patients in creating situations where they can experience being successful. Even small successes (made more likely by breaking long-term goals into small, manageable components) can be powerful motivators as they strengthen an individual's sense of self-efficacy. For instance, it has been found that starting with short bouts of physical activity and gradually working up to longer exercise sessions is more effective than immediately jumping into a full exercise regimen.[47] Talking with patients to identify past situations in which they have experienced success is another strategy for using past experiences to make future attainments more likely.[48]

Some have argued that in cases where performing a particular behavior (such as exercise) *is* objectively possible for the individual, self-efficacy is more appropriately viewed as simply the willingness to perform a behavior. A person can do the behavior if they really want to—that is, if they assume the benefits outweigh the costs associated with the activity.[49, 50] Regardless of whether self-efficacy is simply willingness to try, or something more complicated, the subsequent rewards versus deterrents for various health-related behaviors become the next important step in the behavior-change process.

Perceptions of Benefits and Costs

As illustrated in several of the Chapter 1 models, whether a behavioral change is made and maintained can be determined by perceptions about its costs (e.g., the risks of smoking or the co-pays for prescription medications) as well as benefits (e.g., social gains experienced by hanging out with the boss during "smoking breaks" versus the decreased risk of cancer after quitting). These same concepts of perceived

individual's perceived sense of behavioral control. People with stronger networks of social support feel more empowered to make behavioral changes, and their empowerment enhances their intentions to change, leading ultimately to greater success at achieving their target behaviors.[59]

Psychologists Richard Ryan and Edward Deci argued that social contexts can operate in one of two ways.[60] They can either meaningfully support the development of intrinsic motivation by fostering autonomy and competence, or they can hinder it by exerting control leading to less internalization and integration of behaviors. Thus, motivating others toward commitment and sustained effort should involve supporting their individual efforts and providing an environment in which they can actively practice their skills and improve, rather than simply dictating to them what should or should not be done.

We must note that social support can sometimes be a two-edged sword. One meta-analysis of smoking cessation and partner support found that when partners provided "reminders" in the form of nagging and criticism, smokers were *more* likely to relapse and begin smoking again.[61] This research suggests that when others are involved in a behavioral-change plan, their support should be expressed in non-punitive ways.

Even when members of an individual's social network are not directly involved in a person's behavior change plan, the ongoing pursuit of good health, through adherence and health behavior change, always takes place in a broader social context. There are always both psychosocial costs (barriers) and psychosocial benefits associated with any health behavior. Further, everyone who enacts a new health behavior, consciously or unconsciously, considers and evaluates these elements. In various ways, people assess the complex and often fluctuating interplay of social information, frequently monitoring the costs and benefits of beginning and maintaining goal-directed behavior in the context of social relationships.[62] Such evaluations and adjustments help to assure that balance can be achieved, that the benefits continue to exceed the costs of change, and that motivation, self-efficacy, and commitment are maintained.[63,64]

Goal Framing

As we saw earlier, the way a message about behavior change is framed (presented) can influence its likelihood of adoption. Likewise, framing can also influence whether or not a person stays actively engaged in pursuit of their goal. We previously noted that when individuals compare themselves favorably to others, and perceive that they are increasing in task mastery, they experience higher levels of self-efficacy than if they feel inferior to others and are not improving in their skills. Similarly, research has shown that when people think about their goals as steps toward learning (as opposed to performance indicators) they remain engaged in trying to achieve those goals even following failure.[65] When people frame their goals in terms of increasing their skills, they perceive their own skills more positively and are more likely to be involved in the challenge of behavior change than when they focus on their own performance or on the eventual outcome of their efforts. Thus, the common tendency that many of us have—to focus our attention on the ultimate outcomes of our efforts rather than on the process of acquiring necessary skills—can be a self-defeating strategy. This is especially true when goal-striving behavior must be maintained over time.[66]

Targeting Goals

In this chapter we have presented a lot of information about what might compel someone to take on the challenge of modifying health behaviors and what might engage their continued pursuit of that goal. But, of all the many compelling health goals out there, including eating healthfully, exercising regularly, sleeping enough, and reducing our stress, which ones should we choose to focus on? And how should we make that choice?

It is probably not surprising that, with the exception of unrealistically high goals, setting ambitious aims is likely to result in better outcomes than setting goals that are too easy.[67] Avoiding unrealistically high goals, though, means that the choice of high aims must stay within the realm of things that one is *capable of achieving*.[68,69] Too often, people set for themselves unrealistic health goals (e.g., losing ten pounds by next week). Certainly, television ads for weight-loss programs and for fitness clubs often encourage unrealistic expectations. A more useful strategy, congruent with empirical evidence, involves increasing mastery and learning by setting clear, specific and modest subgoals, involving steps in the bigger process of achieving an ultimate goal.[70] "Lower order" (or stepping-stone) goals allow an individual to build her or his sense of self-efficacy with modest yet measurable achievements, and provide a sense of ongoing mastery and skill refinement.

When setting subgoals, we should remember that there likely exist multiple possible routes to any desired health outcome. For example, achieving a healthy weight can involve various ways of balancing calorie intake and exercise. Plans that allow for more personal choice and that offer individually tailored approaches are likely to be more enjoyable for the individual and are more likely to be maintained over time than rigid programs designed without the specific person in mind.[71] When subgoals are defined and described precisely for the individual, with specific techniques for implementing goal-directed behaviors and the opportunity for modification and adjustment at various points in time, the likelihood of success is increased.[72]

It can be tricky to guide a person toward smaller, achievable goals when she is feeling motivated to take on a bigger and more ambitious task. Telling a patient, "I don't think you'll be able to do that" harms her sense of self-efficacy and is not likely to be productive. Yet, the medical professional may anticipate that the goal as it is currently framed is *not* likely to be something the patient can accomplish. By focusing discussion with the patient on the importance of gaining mastery over

Case Study Box 2.2—Modifying but Not Discouraging Ardis's Goals

At her appointment with Lisa, her health-plan coordinator, Ardis was more upbeat than she'd been in a long time. Attending the weight-loss support group and hearing from people who were even worse off than she was made her feel that her situation wasn't so dire after all. She was now motivated to change! She explained to Lisa that she planned to lose those 70 lbs, and maybe even more, before her college class reunion (which was only 7 months away). She enthusiastically described her plans for going to the gym four times per week, walking every day, and cutting her calorie consumption to about 1,200 per day. Lisa was glad to see Ardis's change in mood and motivation but she could also see that Ardis was setting goals that would be very difficult to achieve. Her challenge now was to direct Ardis's goals appropriately without undermining her sense of self-efficacy.

Lisa: "Ardis, that's wonderful! I'm so glad you found the group to be a helpful resource! I haven't seen you this motivated in a long time, so let's get right down to the specifics. Tell me more about what you'd like to accomplish."

Ardis: "Well, I decided that there's no reason for me to go my class reunion feeling fat and embarrassed about myself. So, I'd like to really work hard and lose those 70 lbs that we've been talking about for so long."

Lisa: "Class reunion, huh? That would motivate me, too! So what have you thought about in terms of specific strategies?"

Ardis: "Well, there's a gym not far from my house and I think I'll buy a membership there. I will be dedicated about it—I'm going to go four times per week, plus I'm going to walk *every* day, and I'm just going to have to cut down on my eating. I was thinking of restricting myself to 1,200 calories per day."

Lisa: "You're an ambitious woman, Ardis. I've found with many of my other patients, though, that a step-up plan that eases you into the larger plan a little more slowly almost always results in better long-term outcomes. I can tell that you're committed to really doing this, so I think an accelerated step-up plan is something you could certainly handle. Shall we go ahead and map out some concrete goals?"

Ardis: "Okay, let's see what that would look like."

                    * * * * * * * * * *

Lisa: "So, let's review what we've got. For the next three days you're going to keep a very detailed record of everything that you eat. Don't try to restrict yourself, just make a note of everything. This will give us a good idea of what your current calorie intake is and will keep us from over-restricting. After you've done that for three days, add them up, take the average, and then reduce your intake by 300 calories per day until our next appointment—that's in two weeks. Okay?"

Ardis: "Three hundred calories doesn't seem like much to cut out."

Lisa: It shouldn't be too hard, you're right. But keep in mind that your body will also be using more calories than it does now, because you're going to be moving more."

Ardis: Right, so I'm going to wear my pedometer all the time and my goal will be 10,000 steps per day for the first two weeks. Doesn't seem hard."

Continued

Lisa: "Yes, you'll be surprised at how easy it is to fit in extra steps here and there. You might also be surprised, though, at how few steps you take now. I remember when I first started wearing a pedometer and my estimates were way off. I thought I probably walked close to 10,000 steps in a day anyway but that first day I only logged 2,700!"

Ardis: "And rather than spending all that money on a gym membership that I might not even use, I'm going to schedule two training sessions with that personal trainer you recommended. She can probably recommend a couple of things for me to buy . . ."

Lisa: "Yes, elastic bands and dumbbells or maybe one of those exercise balls . . . "

Ardis: " . . . and I will do whatever workout she recommends twice per week to start."

Lisa: "I think you've got an excellent plan here. You're going to be practicing some good self-monitoring skills, as well as learning state-of-the-art fitness techniques from that trainer. And in two weeks we'll evaluate things—at that point we'll have a better idea of just how hard we can push you!"

Ardis: "I think you'll be surprised at just how hard I can push *myself*!

---

the process, and by tailoring stepping-stones with the patient's needs and expectations in mind, a plan can be established that maximizes the likelihood of success. The case study box illustrates this for Ardis.

Conclusion

We began this chapter by examining the various factors that contribute to the decision to adopt a goal. These include: upward and downward comparisons; persuasiveness of the argument in favor of a behavior, which is influenced by how much we like and trust the person advocating the behavior; perceptions that an opportunity for change may be lost if a decision is not made; desire to reciprocate good will and to do behaviors that are consistent with each other; and expectations about the likely outcome if a behavior is (or is not) adopted.

We then considered what motivates people to follow up on those choices, actively pursuing their goals and persevering in the struggle to achieve their aims. These factors include: beliefs such as optimism, ability (self-efficacy), and the costs and benefits of acting; social systems that might support behavior change; the size of the goals that are set (e.g., setting subgoals); and the types of goals that are set (e.g., including mastery and skill acquisition as specific goals).

Recognizing that goals cannot be successfully achieved without appropriate information, in Chapter 3 we turn to the topic of how people understand, remember, and recall the information that is important to their health.

References

1. Nagourney E. Insights: possible link between sleep and risk for diabetes. The New York Times. 2008, January 15. Retrieved October 15, 2008 from http://www.nytimes.com/2008/01/15/health/15insi.html?_r=1
2. Eng TR, Maxfield A, Patrick K, Deering MJ, Ratzan SC, Gustafson DH. Access to health information and support: a public highway or a private road? JAMA. 1998 Oct 21;280(15):1371–5.
3. Kenkel DS. Health behavior, health knowledge, and schooling. J Polit Econ. 1991;99(2):287–305.
4. Festinger L. A theory of social comparison processes. Hum Relat. 1954 Oct;7(2):117–40.
5. Buunk BP, Collins RL, Taylor SE, VanYperen NW, Dakof GA. The affective consequences of social comparison: Either direction has its ups and downs. J Pers Soc Psychol. 1990;59(6):1238–49.
6. Helgeson VS, Taylor SE. Social comparisons and adjustment among cardiac patients. J Appl Soc Psychol. 1993;23(15):1171–95.
7. Wills TA. Downward comparison principles in social psychology. Psychol Bull. 1981;90(2):245–71.
8. Gibbons FX. Social comparison as a mediator of response shift. Soc Sci Med. 1999 Jun;48(11):1517–30.
9. Croyle RT. Appraisal of health threats: cognition, motivation, and social comparison. Cognit Ther Res. 1992;16(2):165–82.
10. Buunk BP, Ybema JF. Social comparison and occupational stress: the identification-contrast model. In: Buunk BP, Gibbons FX, editors. Health, Coping and Well-being: Perspectives from Social Comparison Theory. Hillsdale, NJ: Lawrence Erlbaum; 1997. p. 359–88.
11. Van der Zee K, Buunk B, Sanderman R, Botke G, van den Bergh F. Social comparison and coping with cancer treatment. Pers Individ Dif. 2000;28:17–34.
12. Aspinwall LG, Taylor SE. Effects of social comparison direction, threat, and self-esteem on affect, self-evaluation, and expected success. J Pers Soc Psychol. 1993 May;64(5):708–22.
13. Testa M, Major B. The impact of social comparisons after failure: the moderating effects of perceived control. Basic Appl Soc Psychol. 1990;11(2):205–18.
14. Bandura A, Jourden FJ. Self-regulatory mechanisms governing the impact of social comparison on complex decision making. J Pers Soc Psychol. 1991;60(6):941–51.
15. Cialdini RB. Influence: Science and Practice. Boston, MA: Allyn and Bacon; 2001.
16. French J, Raven BH. The basis of social power. In: Cartright D, editor. Studies in Social Power. Ann Arbor, MI: Institute for Social Research; 1959.
17. Rodin J, Janis IL. The social power of health-care practitioners as agents of change. Journal of Social Issues. 1979;35(1):60–81.
18. Buchmann WF. Adherence: a matter of self-efficacy and power. J Adv Nurs. 1997 Jul;26(1):132–7.
19. Eagly AH, Ashmore, Richard D., Makhijani, Mona G., Longo, Laura C. What is beautiful is good, but...: a meta–analytic review of research on the physical attractiveness stereotype. Psychol Bull. 1991; 110(1):109–28.
20. Byrne PS. Evaluation of courses for general practitioners. J R Coll Gen Pract. 1971 Dec;21(113):719–25.

21. Zajonc RB. Attitudinal effects of mere exposure. Journal of Personality and Social Psychology. 1968;35:pp.151–75.
22. Witte K, Allen M. A meta-analysis of fear appeals: implications for effective public health campaigns. Health Educ Behav. 2000 Oct;27(5):591–615.
23. McBride CM, Clipp E, Peterson BL, Lipkus IM, Demark-Wahnefried W. Psychological impact of diagnosis and risk reduction among cancer survivors. Psychooncology. 2000 Sep–Oct;9(5):418–27.
24. Janis IL, Mann L. Effectiveness of emotional role-playing in modifying smoking habits and attitudes. Journal of Experimental Research in Personality. 1965;1:84–90.
25. Mann L, Janis IL. A follow-up study on the long-term effects of emotional role playing. J Pers Soc Psychol. 1968 Apr;8(4):339–42.
26. McBride CM, Emmons KM, Lipkus IM. Understanding the potential of teachable moments: the case of smoking cessation. Health Educ Res. 2003 Apr;18(2):156–70.
27. Rothman AJ, Salovey P. Shaping perceptions to motivate healthy behavior:The role of message framing. Psychol Bull. 1997;121(1):3–19.
28. Wallston KA, Wallston BS, DeVellis R. Development of the Multidimensional Health Locus of Control (MHLC) Scales. Health Educ Monogr. 1978 Spring;6(2):160–70.
29. Shah J. Automatic for the people: how representations of significant others implicitly affect goal pursuit. J Pers Soc Psychol. 2003;84(4):661–81.
30. Besser A, Flett, G.L., & Hewlett, P.L. Perfectionism, cognition, and affect in response to performance failure vs success. Journal of Rational-Emotive & Cognitive Behavior Therapy. 2004;22:301–28.
31. Oishi S, Diener E. Re-examining the general positivity model of subjective well-being: the discrepancy between specific and global domain satisfaction. J Pers. 2001 Aug;69(4):641–66.
32. Sheldon KM, & Kasser, T. Pursuing personal goals: skills enable progress but not all progress is beneficial. Pers Soc Psychol Bull. 1998;24:546–57.
33. Scheier MF, Carver CS. Optimism, coping, and health: assessment and implications of generalized outcome expectancies. Health Psychol. 1985;4(3):219–47.
34. Scheier MF, Carver CS. Effects of optimism on psychological and physical well-being: Theoretical overview and empirical update. Cognit Ther Res. 1992;16(2):201–28.
35. Schwarzer R. Self-regulatory processes in the adoption and maintenance of health behaviors: The role of optimism, goals, and threats. J Health Psychol. 1999;4(2):115–27.
36. Martin LR, Friedman HS, Tucker JS, Tomlinson-Keasey C, Criqui MH, Schwartz JF. A life course perspective on childhood cheerfulness and its relation to mortality risk. Pers Soc Psychol Bull. 2002;28(9):1155–65.
37. Weinstein ND. Unrealistic optimism about susceptibility to health problems: Conclusions from a community-wide sample, J Behav Med. 1987;10(5):481–500.
38. Epstein S. Coping ability, negative self-evaluation, and overgeneralization: experiment and theory. J Pers Soc Psychol. 1992;62(5):826–36.
39. Epstein S, Meier P. Constructive thinking: a broad coping variable with specific components. J Pers Soc Psychol. 1989;57(2):332–50.
40. Ammerman RT, Lynch KG, Donovan JE, Martin CS, Maisto SA. Constructive thinking in adolescents with substance use disorders. Psychol Addict Behav. 2001;15(2):89–96.

41. Park CL, Moore PJ, Turner RA, Adler NE. The roles of constructive thinking and optimism in psychological and behavioral adjustment during pregnancy. J Pers Soc Psychol. 1997;73(3):584–92.
42. Spernak SM, Moore PJ, Hamm LF. Depression, constructive thinking and patient satisfaction in cardiac treatment adherence. Psychol Health Med. 2007;12(2):172–89.
43. Bandura A. Self-efficacy: Toward a unifying theory of behavioral change. Psychol Rev. 1977;84(2):191–215.
44. Stretcher VJ, DeVillis BM, Becker MH, Rosenstock IM. The role of self-efficacy in achieving health behavior change. Health Educ Q. 1986;13(1):73–91.
45. Allison MJ, Keller C. Self-efficacy intervention effect on physical activity in older adults. West J Nurs Res. 2004;26(1):31–46.
46. Luszczynska A, Tryburcy M, Schwarzer R. Improving fruit and vegetable consumption: a self-efficacy intervention compared with a combined self-efficacy and planning intervention. Health Educ Res. 2007 Oct;22(5):630–8.
47. Serdula MK, Khan LK, Dietz WH. Weight loss counseling revisited. JAMA. 2003;289(14): 1747–50.
48. Elder JP, Ayala GX, Harris S. Theories and intervention approaches to health-behavior change in primary care. Am J Prev Med. 1999;17(4):275–84.
49. Kirsch I. Efficacy expectations or response predictions: the meaning of efficacy ratings as a function of task characteristics. J Pers Soc Psychol. 1982;42:132–6.
50. Kirsch I. Response expectancy as a determinant of experience and behavior. Amer Psychol. 1985;4:1189–202.
51. Deci EL, Koestner R, Ryan RM. A meta-analytic review of experiments examining the effects of extrinsic rewards on intrinsic motivation. Psychol Bull. 1999 Nov;125(6):627–68.
52. Rawsthorne LJ, Elliot AJ. Achievement goals and intrinsic motivation: a meta-analytic review. Pers Soc Psychol Rev. 1999;3(4):326–44.
53. Kasser T, Ryan RM. Further examining the American dream: Differential correlates of intrinsic and extrinsic goals. Pers Soc Psychol Bull. 1996;22:80–7.
54. Williams GC, Grow VM, Freedman ZR, Ryan RM, Deci EL. Motivational predictors of weight loss and weight-loss maintenance. J Pers Soc Psychol. 1996 Jan;70(1):115–26.
55. DiMatteo MR. Variations in patients' adherence to medical recommendations: a quantitative review of 50 years of research. Med Care. 2004;42(3):200–9.
56. Fiore MC, Bailey WC, Cohen SJ, Dorfman SF, Goldstein MG, Gritz ER, et al. Treating tobacco use and dependence: clinical practice guideline. Rockville, MD: Department of Health and Human Services, Public Health Service; 2000.
57. Williams GC, McGregor HA, Zeldman A, Freedman ZR, Deci EL. Testing a self-determination theory process model for promoting glycemic control through diabetes self-management. Health Psychol. 2004 Jan;23(1):58–66.
58. Williams GC, Rodin GC, Ryan RM, Grolnick WS, Deci EL. Autonomous regulation and long-term medication adherence in adult outpatients. Health Psychol. 1998 May;17(3):269–76.
59. Courneya KS, McAuley E. Cognitive mediators of the social influence–exercise adherence relationship: A test of the theory of planned behavior. J Behav Med. 1995;18(5):499–515.
60. Ryan RM, Deci EL. Self-determination theory and the facilitation of intrinsic motivation, social development, and well-being. Am Psychol. 2000 Jan;55(1):68–78.

61. Park E, Schultz JK, Tudiver F, Campbell T, Becker L. Enhancing partner support to improve smoking cessation. Cochrane Database Syst Rev. 2002(1):CD002928.
62. Ockene JK, Sorensen G, Kabat-Zinn J, Ockene IS, Donnelly G. Benefits and costs of lifestyle change to reduce risk of chronic disease. Prevent Med. 1988;17(2).
63. O'Dea JA. Why do kids eat healthful food? Perceived benefits of and barriers to healthful eating and physical activity among children and adolescents. J Am Diet Assoc. 2003;103(4):497–551.
64. Zunft HF, Friebe D, Seppelt B, Widhalm K, de Winter AR, Vaz de Almeida MD, Kearney JM, Gibney M. Perceived benefits and barriers to physical activity in a nationally representative sample in the European Union. Public Health Nutr. 2007;2(1):153–60.
65. Elliott ES, Dweck, CS. Goals: An approach to motivation and achievement. J Pers Soc Psychol. 1988;54(1):5–12.
66. Laitakari J, Vuori I, Oja P. Is long-term maintenance of health-related physical activity possible? An analysis of concepts and evidence. Health Educ Res. 1996 Dec;11(4):463–77.
67. Locke EA, Latham GP. Theory of Goal Setting and Task Performance. Englewood Cliffs, NJ: Prentice Hall; 1990.
68. Cervone D, Jiwani N, Wood R. Goal setting and the differential influence of self-regulatory processes on complex decision-making performance. J Pers Soc Psychol. 1991 Aug;61(2):257–66.
69. Locke EA, Frederick E, Lee C, Bobko P. Effect of self-efficacy, goals, and task strategies on task performance. J Appl Psychol. 1984;69:241–51.
70. Strecher VJ, Seijts GH, Kok GJ, Latham GP, Glasgow R, DeVellis B, Meertens RM, Bulger DW. Goal setting as a strategy for health behavior change. Health Educ Q. 1995;22(2):190–200.
71. Dishman RK, Motl RW, Saunders R, Felton G, Ward DS, Dowda M, Pate RR. Enjoyment mediates effects of a school-based physical-activity intervention. Med Sci Sports Exerc. 2005 Mar;37(3):478–87.
72. Gollwitzer PM, Brandstatter V. Implementation intentions and effective goal pursuit. J Pers Soc Psychol. 1997;73(1):186–99.

3

Understanding and Remembering

Everyone has a photographic memory, but not everyone has film.
—Author Unknown

In the seventeenth century, John Locke described the individual as a *tabula rasa* (blank slate) upon which the story of life and of the self would be written. He believed that life experiences not only shaped a person but also set in place the rules by which that shaping would take place. Locke believed that "marks" appear on that slate with the first breath. Many would argue that these marks begin to be etched prenatally, and others even maintain that the slate, even at the very beginning, is never truly blank, but shaped by genetic factors.

The concept of a fresh start—a clean slate—is an appealing notion to many, even later in life after bad habits have been practiced and many mistakes have been made. Many people join gyms and health clubs on January first, vowing to work out five times a week and never eat another donut! Others, such as those with a chronic illness like diabetes, adopt new behavior-change approaches such as a more rigorous testing schedule and maintenance of a record-keeping chart, determined to follow their medical treatment plan faithfully. Some who have been assigned a strict medication regimen work to reorganize their priorities and time in order to remember to take their potentially life-saving pills. The hypertensive patient, for example, may "turn over a new leaf" and set his wristwatch alarm as a reminder—so that he can *finally* be adherent to his treatment. All of these individuals have in common the belief in the possibility of a "fresh start" in changing their behavior.

It is important to remember, of course, that even when starting "fresh," people are *not* "clean slates." Individuals vary in their abilities to plan and to remember, and in their cultural values and norms, personal histories, levels of motivation, beliefs, attitudes, and personalities. These individual differences come together to create *unique slates* on which effective health behaviors can be carved.

In this chapter we will focus primarily on the *information* stage of the Information-Motivation-Strategy model outlined in Chapter 1 in order to evaluate

51

the issues of understanding and remembering as they relate to health behavior change.

Information Processing, Memory, and Recall

Let's begin this section with a few basic, and necessarily oversimplified, facts about how memory works. The process of memory can be divided into three essential components: encoding, storage, and retrieval. *Encoding* refers to the process of putting information into memory, and it requires effort. We simply don't remember things that we don't notice or pay attention to; encoding requires attention to whatever is to be remembered. *Storage* involves the maintenance of information in memory over time. Memory is increasingly understood as a dynamic and constructive process, rather than as a static entity; "pure" memory is likely very rare. Instead, studies show that memories can change over time, as elements of memory for some events degrade and others are continuously integrated with new information or older, "cross-over" data. *Retrieval* refers to the process of recalling information that has been stored and integrated, bringing it back into conscious awareness.

Sometimes a stored memory is difficult to retrieve; it feels close to awareness, but can't quite be accessed. This is called the "tip-of-the-tongue phenomenon."[1] When we successfully recall a stored memory, we experience the aspect of memory process that most people think of as "memory"—but, it's easy to forget that there are several steps that precede this one! Let's examine these preliminary steps in more detail.

Focusing Attention and Encoding

The first step in the memory process involves noticing and paying attention to something. Largely without even thinking about it, we all filter information and focus on, or "attend" to, particular things, ignoring others. If we didn't, we would be quickly overwhelmed by the sheer volume of incoming information! By focusing attention on something, we can make it part of our short-term or "working" memory. But, we also do not focus attention randomly—we direct attention to things that are important to us, and tend to notice things that are consistent with our preexisting ideas and expectations.

Our immediate, or short-term memory, is quite limited; most people are only able to store about seven things there at once. In computer terms, short-term memory is analogous to RAM (random access memory) which is used for active processing of information in real time and which is being constantly "written over"; this is contrasted with long-term memory, similar to a computer's ROM (read-only memory), which is the much larger capacity to store information permanently. The things that we actively use in working memory may include those that are occurring right now as well as older information that we bring into consciousness in order to help us solve a problem we are currently working on.[2] For older adults (about ages 61 to 80) in particular, understanding and memory for information that is presented rapidly[3] and that requires more processing in working memory[4] can be poorer than it is for younger persons (about ages 17 to 32). This is important, because much of what is presented to patients during medical visits is both fast-paced and complex. Thus, the fact that old age is often a negative predictor of memory performance is accentuated in situations such as these, where demands on working memory are high. Issues of working memory are particularly relevant to the process of adhering to treatment. At home, a person might "remember" to take their medication but then fail to actually do so because they are distracted by a ringing phone, a sick dog, or an intrusive memory about some other task that had been momentarily forgotten. These intrusions to working memory might effectively push out what had been the person's focus: to get that pill and take it, leaving him or her wondering, "Now, why did I come into the kitchen?" With practice, rehearsal, and sometimes the use of memory-enhancing strategies (which we discuss later in the chapter), information can be maintained at the forefront of attention until a task is completed, or moved from short-term, working memory to long-term storage, where the capacity is believed to be limitless.

Memory Storage

Studies have shown that memory is not stored in a single, particular *place* in the brain. For example, when rats have learned to navigate a maze, there is no single area of the brain that, when destroyed, will render them unable to complete the maze.[5] Research also demonstrates that ongoing electrical activity in the brain is *not* required for memory to be maintained. Rats and hamsters that were taught to navigate a maze were then cooled so that all brain activity stopped; after they were revived they could still complete the maze just fine.[6, 7]

Instead, memory involves a process called long-term potentiation (LTP) in which certain neural pathways become strengthened through activity. This is somewhat like the neurons developing "habits" in the ways they communicate with each other. We also know that certain neurotransmitters influence the ease with which these "habits" are formed.

Another fascinating fact about the brain is its "plasticity." This means that different areas of the brain can take over the types of tasks and memory storage that were once done by other parts if those parts should be damaged, such as in the case of a traumatic brain injury or a stroke. Findings such as these give us insights into the memory processes that can be important to achieving health behavior change.

Emotion and Memory

Have you ever noticed that some things seem to be etched in your memory from the moment of experience? Or that some memories seem so much more vivid to you than others? Researchers believe that this is partly due to the emotional content of the experience. The concept "flashbulb memory" describes such a memory that is so emotionally intense and significant that it is remembered in great detail.[8] For example, you may remember exactly where you were and what you were doing when you first heard about the terrorist attacks that took place on September 11, 2001. This involves the idea of flashbulb memory. When experiences are emotionally charged, the brain's *amygdaloid complex* is more active,[9] and it appears that this area of the brain interacts over the short term with stress hormones to regulate the strength of stored memories according to their emotional potency (i.e., their importance).[10, 11]

This may be good news for health behavior change. Receiving information about a serious health threat will no doubt be emotional for most individuals; in this way, emotion can enhance memory by making events more salient. However, if an emotion is extremely intense—especially if it is threatening—it can overwhelm a person's senses and interfere with encoding. Thus, most people are unlikely to forget a diagnosis (although they might forget its technical name), but they often do forget what they are supposed to do to treat or manage it. When people receive a diagnosis, they are typically upset and their heightened emotional state can be detrimental to the encoding of treatment information that they are subsequently given. In this case, memory of the moment when the problematic test results were first heard may be quite clear, but the associated distress may interfere with the person's ability to focus on and encode treatment instructions and information about follow-up.[12]

One series of studies demonstrated that when the content of a message was emotionally charged, a simple main point seemed to be remembered well, but memory for the surrounding information was impaired by the emotional content.[13] Health professionals must keep this in mind in order to strategically influence their patients' abilities to attend to and remember the crucial information that follows distressing medical information. This may be accomplished by using effective communication strategies and providing reassurance to patients. Some principles for helping patients remember medical information are summarized in Table 3.1.

Although an emotionally charged diagnosis has the potential to make encoding, storage, and recall of follow-up medical information more difficult, clearly linking the diagnosis to the recommendations that follow can minimize this barrier. For example, one study demonstrated that when patients had a disease that could be managed with effective health-behavior changes, and it was emphasized that the health promotion advice they received would help them to make these changes, the patient's recall was twice as good as it was when the same health behavior advice was provided but not directly related to the diagnosis.[14] This finding might be expanded to imply that if health *risks* can be made salient to patients, and those risks (and their reduction) are clearly linked to health behavior recommendations, those recommendations might be remembered quite well.

If the patient's level of anxiety or fear in response to the news is too high, however, it is possible that he or she may simply "tune out," believing (often

Table 3.1 What health professionals can do to help patients remember medical information.

1. Speak slowly and don't rush through the information you are providing to the patient
2. Refrain from using medical jargon
3. Even if you think you have not used jargon, check frequently to make sure the patient understood your meaning
4. Know the patient's level of health literacy and convey information at an appropriate level
5. Understand that patients receiving a diagnosis may be upset and emotional and this may impede their ability to remember treatment and follow-up information
6. Provide comfort and reassurance to patients to alleviate anxiety and increase capacity to attend and remember
7. Pair health-behavior change information with other meaningful information (a related diagnosis, for example)
8. Be aware of patients' health beliefs
9. Tailor and personalize information that is given to patients
10. Don't give too much information at once
11. Put the most important information first and last
12. Encourage patients to take notes
13. Suggest, or provide, memory aids (written materials, illustrations, mnemonics, etc.)

incorrectly) that the disease has progressed too far and that nothing can be done.[15] Clearly, the time of diagnosis may represent a teachable moment, as discussed in the last chapter, but the patient's anxiety must be managed so that this moment is not lost. As we noted in Chapter 2, the emotion generated by the diagnosis must not be so overwhelming as to incapacitate the patient, and clear steps to ameliorate the negative possibilities must be provided so that the patient can effectively understand and remember the necessary steps to self-management.

Chronic Stress

In addition to interfering with attention and focus, stress can actually affect physiological functioning in such a way as to affect memory. With long-term stress (such as over the course of an illness or a set of life problems, rather than associated with the momentary arousal of receiving bad news), the presence of associated glucocorticoids can interfere with cognitive processing and memory, in part by causing atrophy of the part of the brain called the hippocampus.[10, 16, 17] Thus, people who struggle with the stresses of a serious disease over time may have increasing difficulty remembering essential elements of their treatment plan. This may explain, in part, one of the interesting findings to come out of a recent meta-analysis. Treatment adherence among patients with serious diseases was actually worse when patients were more, compared with less, severely ill.[18] Patients such as these may need additional help to remember the behaviors they are to carry out, especially if changes are made to an already-familiar treatment regimen.

Self-Enhancement Bias

Despite the fact that the emotion associated with "bad news" can be easily recalled, research shows that the actual content of people's recollections often tends to be affected by self-enhancement bias. That is, people generally tend to remember things with a positive bias, actually believing things are better or that they are healthier than they really are. In one study, it was the people who received the worst results from their tests of cholesterol and cardiovascular risk who were most likely to recall, several months later, that their results were better than they actually had been. Thus, those with the worst health-risk profiles engaged in the most self-enhancing memory bias, thinking of themselves as healthier than they really were.[19]

Similarly, when information about health behavior is particularly disturbing (e.g., that a person is exercising far less than ideal), research shows that instead of improving the behavior, the individual is likely to minimize stress by changing his or her views about the behavior.[20] This is consistent with what the theory of cognitive dissonance would predict—it suggests that people are driven to seek consistency in their attitudes and behaviors, and to frequently change attitudes to make them consistent with behaviors.[21] For example, Ryan has been trying to increase his physical activity for nearly two years, with little success. Alice (the physician's assistant whom he sees regularly) notes that his concept of how much exercise he needs to do and what constitutes exercise has changed rather dramatically over the past six months. He doesn't see his sedentary practices as particularly disturbing, citing that he walks quite a bit and giving "walking from the car to the store" and "vacuuming" as evidence. Although these behaviors can be an important part of an active lifestyle, they are not enough to fulfill Ryan's physical activity requirements. Ryan seems not to be able to see this, however. Alice decides that she will spend some time during their next visit comparing with Ryan his activity levels of two years ago with his current level and the ideal. She hopes to help him see how his own thinking has changed. She also puts a note in his chart requesting that his physician provide as much information as possible about Ryan's downward progression and its associated risks during their next visit; she believes that raising Ryan's anxiety about his health may prompt him to take action to change.

Cultural Context

Several quite prominent and stable qualities of individual identity also tend to influence memory. These features, such as ethnicity, religion, family, and other cultural influences, need to be understood and considered during the medical encounter, although they are not likely to be changed. In Chapter 1 we examined the importance of beliefs to health behavior change; as we further explore memory, we can begin to understand the pervasive effects of these beliefs, through the mechanism of culture.

Beliefs are maintained, in part, through the process of "cognitive filtering." This means that we generally tend to notice and be more attentive to information that confirms what we already believe to be true (keep in mind that people attend to less than 1 percent of the information in their visual fields!), often ignoring or discounting contradictory information altogether.[22] We also tend to interpret ambiguous things in a way that is consistent with what we already think we know[23] and we do not assign equal weight to all incoming information. Instead, we tend to put more weight on information that is important to us and consistent with our preconceptions.[24–26] The dramatic differences in understanding that this cognitive filtering process can create is illustrated in the case study box.

Case Study Box 3.1—The Influence of Cognitive Filters on Understanding in the Medical Visit

Ron and Don are both patients of Dr. François. They both have diabetes and are similar in terms of their disease progression. Their backgrounds are quite different, however, and this plays an important role in their understanding of what Dr. François tells them.

Don grew up in a family where being responsible and take-charge was valued; Ron's family tended to encourage a "go with the flow" approach. Don's family emphasized eating healthfully and keeping fit. Special occasions in Ron's family centered around eating, and no efforts were ever made to cook healthy meals. Both of Don's parents went to college and he and his siblings were always taught the value of scientific findings. Nobody in Ron's family has gone to college and there is a tendency to be suspicious of science among Ron's family and peers. Don recognizes that diabetes is a serious illness; Ron believes that diabetes is really no big deal—he knows quite a few people who have it and they seem to get along just fine.

What Dr. François says: "You're going to have to be especially careful around the holidays if you want to keep your blood sugar within the target range."
What Don interprets: "I'm going to have to use extra willpower during the holidays; if I want to have something special at a party or gathering I'd better compensate for it with a brisk walk afterwards or by eating a little differently before I go to the event."
What Ron interprets: "I've been doing well with keeping my blood sugar within the limits. If I slip up a little during the holidays, that's ok, so long as I stick to my diet at least part of the time. That will be better than I did last year."
What Dr. François says: "I see here that we're missing a few entries on your blood glucose record sheet for tests this month."

Continued

What Don interprets: "She's disappointed in me for not being as conscientious as I should with my testing. I am going to make sure not to miss any more tests, and to write them down as soon as I've taken them."

What Ron interprets: "She seems glad that I've got most of my entries recorded. I wonder if now she'll let me slack off a little on the number of times I have to do those finger pricks."

What Dr. François says: "I believe I see some small changes in your left retina as compared to a few months ago. It's difficult to tell, so I'd like to refer you to a specialist for a more careful look."

What Don interprets: "Despite the fact that I've been doing pretty well at regulating my diet, I'm still not maintaining my visual health! There's still lots of room for improvement in my behaviors and I need to make some serious changes if I want to maintain my eyesight."

What Ron interprets: "Another eye exam . . . ok, if I have time. Maybe after the holidays. I'm sure everyone's eyes go through small changes all the time anyway, so it doesn't sound very serious."

Besides filtering out (or accentuating) parts of the communicative exchange, cultural factors also play an important role in a person's willingness to engage a health message and the ease with which health behaviors can be changed. One's family history, for example, may have ingrained an active orientation toward illness. A person with this inclination is likely to listen carefully as a risk factor is described or a diagnosis is made, and then tackle the challenge of disease management head-on. Aspects of the current family environment (e.g., being married and thus having someone else encouraging positive health behaviors) may also influence the degree to which an individual attends to health-related messages.[27] If dietary recommendations are dramatically different from an individual's cultural norms (and especially if important social interactions center around these cultural dishes), a person might be quite resistant to dietary change. If there are strong pressures on a patient to use "natural, herbal" remedies that have been in the family for generations rather than relying on pills prescribed by a doctor, adherence to a medication regimen may be much more difficult.

Thus, aspects of one's own culture and personal history not only play a role in the process of attending to health information and initially encoding it, but may also predict the amount of work the individual is willing or feels able to do in order to remember and act on health-related information.

Additional Factors

Some of the factors that people commonly associate with memory really do not seem to make much difference. For example, although some studies find that women's memory for personally experienced events tends to be better than men's, other kinds of memory (such as for verbal information) have not been found to differ between the sexes.[28, 29] Other assumptions about memory, however, contain at least a kernel of truth. Despite individual variations, old age is a fairly reliable negative predictor of memory,[30] although the effects vary for different kinds of memory. Memory for specific content seems less influenced by age than is contextual information,[31] and, as we noted earlier, rapid presentation and high demands on working memory are also more problematic for older adults.[3, 4]

Health professionals should keep in mind issues of memory, particularly when working with older patients. Consider the nurse practitioner, Allison, who makes a conscious effort not to rush too quickly when she makes her weekly phone calls to 85-year-old Peter. Her queries about his blood glucose, blood pressure, and sodium intake (all of which he manages for himself) are typically made in the same order. She consciously tries to offer a patterned familiarity to their conversations. She also encourages him to make notes to himself and to write down the date and hour each time he takes his medications. This helps him not only to remember to take his prescriptions, but keeps him from taking double-doses.

Transient characteristics, such as sleep-deprivation or substance use can also play a crucial role in memory. Although the direct links between sleep deprivation and the ability to establish new memory traces are not yet clear in research, sleep deprivation is consistently associated with a variety of cognitive ill effects including difficulty concentrating.[32, 33] Because attention is critically important for encoding memory, interference with attention is likely to indirectly affect memory itself. In addition, research demonstrates that for a variety of types of tasks and experiences, remembering, recall, and task performance are better when those tasks or experiences are followed by sleep.[34, 35] It seems that new memory traces, which tend to be relatively fragile, are reactivated and strengthened during sleep and the traces are better translated into long-term memories.[36, 37] Thus, a person who is sleep deprived may have difficulty concentrating on what goes on during a medical visit, and may also tend to forget much of what they had initially retained if their memory traces are not solidified during subsequent periods of adequate sleep.

In a similar way, drugs (including alcohol and even some prescribed medications) can impair an individual's initial ability to focus on and appropriately attend to what is happening during a medical interaction. These substances may also hinder memory consolidation through several different cognitive processes and pathways.[11]

Another transient (and changeable) factor influencing memory and recall is the length of the medical visit itself. Studies suggest that in longer, as opposed to briefer, medical visits patients have a greater chance of recalling the information presented to them.[14] How long is long enough? Researchers believe that at least 19 minutes may be essential to ensure enough time for true patient participation, information sharing, and fully answering patients' questions.[38] In cases where 19 minutes is impossible, making effective use of whatever time is available becomes even more crucial. Let's turn now to some strategies that might be used to help patients remember.

Strategies for Improving Memory and Recall

Tailoring Information

It is still common to find, in various healthcare settings, "one size fits all" informational pamphlets that provide the reader with general information about a disease condition and some helpful strategies to combat it. Although these can sometimes be useful, they are often too general to be of much help. It is also easier for patients to discount this type of communication, rationalizing that it's mass-produced and not really "designed for me."

Today's technology makes it relatively simple to create information sheets, directives, and other health-relevant behavior plans that are specifically tailored to individuals. For example, physical therapists frequently employ computer programs with data banks of pictures and instructions for various exercises. They create and print out sets of exercises designed to address a patient's individual needs. Similarly, a registered dietitian may provide individualized counseling to patients, helping them to develop a personalized meal plan that suits their unique nutritional needs and food preferences. Even if there are no preexisting data banks for a particular illness, disease, or injury, healthcare professionals may choose to create their own with techniques, exercises, diet plans, or tips that they use frequently with their patient populations. As their own data bases develop, they are able to more efficiently tailor the materials that accompany the verbal medical advice they give to their patients.

Research shows that people take tailored information such as this more seriously than general information. They are more likely to read information that is put together especially for them; they find it more interesting, they remember it better, and they are more likely to save the paperwork for future reference.[39–41] A theoretical model by Petty and Cacioppo[42] called the Elaboration Likelihood Model (ELM) proposes that additionally, tailored messages tend to prompt people to engage more thoughtfully with the material than they would with general messages, resulting in more effective behavior change. Of course, if a message created to promote behavior change in a larger group of people happens to fit the individual very well, it is likely to have the same impact as a message specifically tailored to the person,[43] but this often does not happen.

It is also important to note that a tailored message is likely to interact with an individual's characteristics, such as self-efficacy for behavior change. One study, for example, found that for people with high self-efficacy, a tailored message regarding weight loss was more effective than was a generic message. On the other hand, this study found that those with low self-efficacy (who thought they could not change) responded more negatively to a tailored message than to a general message. They tended to feel threatened and to generate counterarguments to the points of the message.[44] This represents one more case in which knowing more about the patient (this time, his or her beliefs about personal ability) allows for more effective targeting of a message. For a patient with high self-efficacy, a tailored message will likely work well; for a patient with low self-efficacy, care should be taken to modify the message to be as nonthreatening and as encouraging as possible.

When tailored messages are unavailable, or for other reasons are impractical, general information should still be given, but only *following* a discussion of the personalized issue or problem (e.g., after the patient's diagnosis is discussed with her or him). This makes patients more likely to feel that the general information they receive is important and that their health professional means it specifically for them.[45] The importance of a verbal health message is highlighted if it is accompanied by a written prescription (such as for exercise)[46] and this prescription can then be paired with the informational pamphlet, making the general information more personally relevant.

Dr. Bueller's office has instituted a method for personalizing "general" health information pamphlets by including a checklist of available informational materials in each patient's chart. After each visit, Dr. Bueller hands the chart to her receptionist, Julie, for scheduling the next appointment. At the counter near the door out to the waiting room, Julie can easily initiate a private conversation like the following:

Julie: Ok, Mrs. Jones, we've got you set for your follow-up appointment next Thursday. Here's a reminder card for that—I've got the time written on there for you, as well.

Mrs. Jones: Good, thank you.

Julie: Now, here is something else that Dr. Bueller wanted me to give you. This is a pamphlet that has some tips for decreasing sodium in your diet, and even has a couple of good recipes. Dr. Bueller would like you to have this—she thinks it might help you make some of the dietary changes you two have been talking about. Ok?

This follow-up to a topic that has been brought up (even briefly) by the physician during the medical encounter, is likely to be much more effective than simply having the receptionist give out pamphlets in the absence of physician-initiated discussion of the topic (or having the pamphlets available in a waiting-room display). Patients are more likely to remember to read the information if it is specifically given to them; and, because they attend to it better, they are also more likely to retain it.

Making Time

As we have seen, when health-care professionals present information in visits that are not rushed, patients tend to remember better. Thus, one effective strategy is simply to schedule adequate time for the medical visit. Health professionals should allow enough time for patients to actively engage, to ask questions, and to understand what it is that they need to do. If physicians cannot take as much time as the patient needs, nurses or other members of the health-care team should be available to help them. Studies show that time spent with other members of the health-care team can be just as effective as time spent with the primary care doctor.[47]

Although this is a simple and straightforward strategy, it is not always easy to accomplish. Patients who want more time typically find that this is not under their direct control, and even physicians report that they do not have as much time to spend with their patients as they would prefer.[48, 49] From the patient's side, it is worth being assertive and asking for some time for health behavior education from a member of the physician's staff. Given what we know about attention and memory, patients can make sure they make good use of the time allocated for their visits by coming to their appointments well rested and prepared with any questions they might have. This can be encouraged by the health-care professional at the time the appointment is made and in any reminder phone calls or mailings that are done. Patients are routinely reminded about other sorts of preparations, such as not eating or drinking anything but water for a period of time before a fasting blood test. Expanding suggested preparation to include adequate rest beforehand, and thoughts about what they hope to achieve in the visit, will aid the patient's ability to concentrate and focus on the medical exchange.

Avoiding Overload

Research data clearly indicate that as more information is presented to patients, they forget a larger proportion of it.[50–52] For this reason it is especially important that patients not be overloaded with too much information; they will feel overwhelmed and will fail to remember it all.

In addition, patients must understand what it is that they are to remember, before they can hope to actually store and then recall it.[53, 54] So, in addition to avoiding volume overload (too much information) we must also think about complexity overload (information that is too complicated). We know from numerous studies that patients are not very likely to actively assert their need for clarification or to ask a lot of questions when they don't understand something.[55, 56] This highlights the importance of taking a patient's health literacy into account, providing information at a level that is appropriate for each patient's understanding, and using language that is as straightforward and as jargon-free as possible.[57–59]

The term *health literacy* refers to an individual's ability to obtain and understand the basic health information that is relevant to her or his situation.[60–62] Although health literacy is correlated with general education,[63] it is not the case that well-educated or smart people are always health literate! Some very intelligent people might know little, or have some inaccurate beliefs, about health.

Despite individual variations, studies show, however, that physicians generally tend to overestimate their patients' levels of knowledge[64] and to use terms and descriptions that their patients often don't have the health literacy to interpret correctly. For health professionals, medical jargon comes easily to the tongue—it is comfortable and familiar, it is precise, and what can be described in medical terms with just a word or two may require a detailed and lengthy explanation in everyday language. Nonetheless, it is important to resist the temptation to speak to patients in "med-speak." For example, one study found that patients are correct in their understanding of medical terms only about 36% of the time.[57] In another study in which 71 percent of participants were college-educated, respondents were asked to define 50 general medical terms; none of these terms was correctly identified by everyone and only 10 participants (out of 224) correctly defined all the terms.[65] See Table 3.2 for a listing of some of the incorrect definitions for medical terms that were identified in classic studies of jargon.[66, 67]

It is impossible to know, based on things like age or education level, exactly how health literate a person is. Formal assessments of a patient's level of health literacy can thus be very helpful in appropriately targeting information to the individual's level of comprehension.[68, 69] It may be instructive, for example, for patients to complete brief health literacy screenings and for physicians and other health-care professionals to have access to this information in the patients' chart. The providers can then know when to use simpler language or provide printed materials that are designed for low–health literacy patients.[70] Or, for patients with greater health literacy, more information may be given, or information that the patient already understands well may be touched on only briefly so as to leave more time to discuss the areas that the patient is less familiar with. The case study box provides an illustration of how a discussion about diabetes management might be quite different for a patient with low versus high health literacy.

To ensure that understanding has actually been achieved, patients should also repeat back to the health-care professional in their own words (known as the "teach-back" method) the most crucial elements of what they need to know.[71] This not only demonstrates understanding (and provides the opportunity for the clinician to clarify or make corrections if there are any misunderstandings), but it also aids the patient as she or he begins to consolidate that information into memory.[68]

Table 3.2 Some classic misinterpretations of medical terms.

Abdomen	Sides; buttocks; back; uterus; heart; bladder; area below the waist
Appendectomy	Rupture of the appendix; pain in the stomach; cut rectum; taking off an arm or leg; something like an epidemic; something to do with the bowels
Incubation period	Being hospitalized and put into an incubator
Intern	Someone that helps in the hospital; same as an orderly; a male nurse; a doctor without a degree

Case Study Box 3.2—Two Sample Explanations of a Pulmonary Function Test Targeted for a Patient with Low versus High Health Literacy

Low Health Literacy

"Good Morning, Mrs. Malcolm. Today we're going to work on figuring out why you've been so short of breath lately—why you feel out-of-breath even when you're not doing anything much. Do you have any questions before we get started?" (Patient responds that she does not.)

"Okay, I'm going to have you sit right here, and put this clip on your nose like this. This is to make sure that all your breathing is done through your mouth so we can get an accurate reading with this machine. Now, this tube goes into your mouth, you can grip it with your teeth if you like, but be sure to close your lips around it so that no air escapes when you breathe out. I'm going to ask you to take a nice, deep breath, and then you are going to breathe out as hard as you can. While you're breathing out I'll count to six, and it's important that you keep breathing out until I get to six, ok? Even if you feel like you're out of air, try to keep pushing more air out through the tube until you hear me say 'six', alright?" (Patient responds in the affirmative, and completes the first exhalation as instructed.)

"Ok, Mrs. Malcolm, that was good. The machine gives me a reading of how much air you were able to force out. Now, we're going to do exactly the same thing two more times, and we'll take the best one—whichever one shows the most air being forced out of your lungs, ok?" (Patient responds in the affirmative and the next two exhalations are completed.)

"That was great, Mrs. Malcolm. We're all done with that now. Let me get these printouts, and we'll talk about what we're going to do next."

High Health Literacy

"Good morning Mrs. Elias. Today we're going to be doing a pulmonary function test with you, trying to Figure out what's going on with your lungs that's making you short of breath lately. Do you have any questions before we get started?" (Patient responds that she does not.)

"Ok, I'm going to have you sit right here, and put this clip on your nose. Now, in just a minute this tube will go into your mouth, be sure to create an air-tight seal with your lips so that no air escapes when you exhale. The air you exhale is going into this machine and it's going to show us how much air volume you can move in and out of your lungs— that's called your "forced vital capacity" and how fast you can move that air. I'm going to ask you to take a nice, deep breath, and then you are going to breathe out as hard as you can. While you're breathing out I'll count to six, and it's important that you keep breathing out until I get to six, ok? Even if you feel like you're out of air, try to keep pushing more air out through the tube until you hear me say 'six', alright?" (Patient responds in the affirmative.)

"We're going to go through the whole inhalation-exhalation process three times, and we'll evaluate the best one. Any questions?" (Patient responds that she does not, and completes all three exhalations as instructed.)

Ok, Mrs. Elias, that was great. Let me grab these printouts. We're going to compare your performance with the normal values for someone of your age, gender, body size, and

> **Continued**
>
> ethnicity—all of which influence what is considered "normal" lung functioning. This will give us some idea of what might be causing your shortness of breath, for starters whether your airflow is restricted or obstructed. How does that sound?"

Ordering of Information

A well-known finding from the learning and memory literature is that people tend to remember best the first and the last things that a speaker presents. These tendencies are called *primacy effects* (remembering the first thing) and *recency effects* (remembering the last thing).[72] This quirk of memory can be used as a tool by the astute clinician who places the most crucial pieces of information at the beginning and the end of the visit. In addition to aiding recall, this placement also emphasizes the importance of those particular pieces of information, since it has been shown that patients tend to view as most important the things they hear first.[50]

Note-Taking and Memory Aids

Encouraging patients to make notes before and during their medical visits can be one of the most reliable methods for improving their ability to participate in their own medical care and their success in recalling the details of their medical visit. In fact, the medical office itself is an ideal place to provide materials that patients can use to write down their questions (perhaps small notepads in the waiting room or the exam room, for instance). The medical office can also provide other memory aids, in the form of alternative media, that can facilitate patients' understanding and recall of medical information.

Alternative media (i.e., something other than just written material) may be one of the most effective prompts for those whose reading and writing skills are not top-notch. A substantial segment of the population falls into this category; one large-scale study in the United States identified 23 percent of English-speaking and 34 percent of Spanish-speaking patients as unable to read and understand medical information presented in their primary spoken language.[73] Another study estimates an eighth- or ninth-grade reading level for the average adult in the United States,[74] yet many health-care directives are written at or above the tenth grade level,[75] and many HIPAA notices and surgical informed-consent documents use language appropriate for the college graduate level.[76, 77]

Considering these challenges, it makes sense to supplement verbal information and instructions with illustrative materials that the patient can take home; and research shows that this can be quite effective. A recent review of the utility of using visual aids, for example, found that pairing pictures and illustrations with verbal content increases both attention to educational material and later recall of the material.[78] These effects can be dramatic, with one study increasing recall from just 15 to 85 percent using this picture-pairing method [79] Simple pictures such as cartoon or line drawings seemed to aid comprehension and recall better than detailed, shaded drawings or photographs[80, 81] probably because they provide fewer distracting details. This is good news, since simple drawings are easier to produce and can even be created in-house without much difficulty. Figure 3.1 provides an example of how instructions for taking medications might be illustrated—note that *both* words and illustrations are used, which has been shown by the research to be most effective.

As we noted previously, any written or alternative media materials (e.g., informational pamphlets, instructional DVDs) should be tailored to the individual or at least appropriately targeted to specifics of the patient's case in order to be most helpful. If illustrations reflect individuals that are similar to the patient (e.g., same

Eat breakfast first thing in the morning, than wait 2 hours.

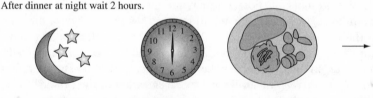

After 2 hours, take 2 pills with 2 glasses of water.

After dinner at night wait 2 hours.

Then take 1 pill with 2 glasses of Water.

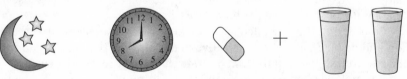

Figure 3.1 Illustration of medication instructions supplemented by drawings.

ethnicity) this tends to be preferred by patients [82, 83] and may also result in better comprehension of the material.[84]

Illustrations and visual aids cannot take the place of verbal instruction, however. They are meant to be supplemental, not a substitution. When a picture is used to integrate information that the patient doesn't understand in the first place, it is useless. In fact, it may be worse than useless because the patient may use the picture to try to guess what they are supposed to do, and they may guess incorrectly.[85] Thus, illustrations should be used as tools to reinforce and further explain what is already part of the medical communication, and should be selected to fit with the patient's level of health literacy.

Mnemonics and Chunking

Other memory aids include using mnemonics (phrases or acronyms that represent important elements of what must be remembered) or chunking (organizing information into more manageable groups or chunks). Although the clinician will probably not have much time to spend going over such memory strategies with patients, these tools can be quite effective when applied to self-directed behavior change, and their utility is reinforced when health-care personnel advocate their use. And, they can be especially helpful for patients who aren't taking notes but need to remember a list or sequence of behaviors. For example, an eye-catching poster with illustrations of a series of behaviors may be more easily recalled than a mere verbal description of the list.[78] One useful acronym, this one for helping patients remember the steps they should take to actively participate in their own health care is PREPARED®.[86, 87] PREPARED® is a framework for communication between health-care professionals and patients that encourages patients to ask questions and be involved in making health-care decisions. This memory aid, along with other sample acronyms, can be found in Table 3.3.

Table 3.3 Examples of acronyms for prompting recall of medically relevant behaviors.

PREPARED®
Aids patients in participatory decision-making

Prescription or Procedure—What is the recommended treatment?
Reason—What is the reason for undergoing this treatment?
Expectation—What are the expectations for the treatment?
Probability—What is the likelihood the treatment will be effective?
Alternatives—What are alternatives to this recommended treatment?
Risks—What are the risks of the recommended treatment?
Expenses—What are the financial or other costs of the treatment?
Decision—Based on the answers to the previous questions, what is the decision about the treatment?

(Continued)

Table 3.3 (Continued)

ICE
Initial treatment for a strain, sprain, or contusion

Ice should be applied for 20 minutes to help reduce pain and swelling
Compression should be applied to help reduce swelling
Elevation of the injured area can also help reduce swelling

ADHERE[88]
Promotes adherence to treatment regimens

Assess readiness for treatment
Determine health goals and priorities
Help with implementation
Elicit feedback
Review adherence measures
Evaluate effectiveness

Conclusion

In this chapter we have explored a number of strategies for helping patients to understand their medical issues and remember what it is that they are supposed to do. These included things like using tailored messages, taking time and explaining clearly, providing illustrations and alternative media to complement verbal and written instructions, and using other memory aids such as mnemonics and the strategy of chunking information. But of course using all of these tools to increase understanding and memory doesn't assure that patients will take action regarding the things they have learned. The transition between knowing what should be done and actually making those behaviors habitual is the focus of our next chapter. In Chapter 4 we explore the strengths, weaknesses, and skills that each person brings to the behavior change challenge, and the strategies that individuals can employ to maximize their health-behavior change success.

References

1. Schwartz BL. Tip-of-the-tongue states: phenomenology, mechanism, and lexical retrieval. Metacognition and Learning. 2002;1(2):149–58.
2. Engle RW. Working memory capacity as executive attention. Current Directions in Psychological Science. 2002;11:19–23.
3. Stine EL, Wingfield A, Poon LW. How much and how fast: rapid processing of spoken language in later adulthood. Psychol Aging. 1986 Dec;1(4):303–11.
4. Kemper S. Geriatric psycholinguistics: syntactic limitations of oral and written language. In: Light L, Burke D, editors. Language, Memory, and Aging. New York: Cambridge University Press; 1988. p. 58–76.

5. Lahley KS. In search of the engram. Symposium of the Society for Experimental Biology. New York: Cambridge University Press; 1950.
6. Andjus RK, Knopfelmacher F, Russell RW, Smith AU. Some effects of severe hypothermia on learning and retention. The Quarterly Journal of Experimental Psychology. 1956;8:15–23.
7. Gerard RW. What Is Memory? New York: Freeman; 1953.
8. Brown R, Kulik J. Flashbulb memory. Cognition. 1977;5:73–99.
9. Cahill L, Haier RJ, Fallon J, Alkire MT, Tang C, Keator D, Wu J, McGaugh JL. Amygdala activity at encoding correlated with long-term, free recall of emotional information. Proc Natl Acad Sci USA. 1996 Jul 23;93(15):8016–21.
10. McEwen BS, Sapolsky RM. Stress and cognitive function. Curr Opin Neurobiol. 1995 Apr;5(2):205–16.
11. McGaugh JL. Memory consolidation and the amygdala: a systems perspective. Trends Neurosci. 2002 Sep;25(9):456.
12. Kessels RP. Patients' memory for medical information. J R Soc Med. 2003 May;96(5):219–22.
13. Christianson SA, Loftus EF. Remembering emotional events: the fate of detailed information. Cogn Emot. 1991;5(2):81–108.
14. Flocke SA, Stange KC. Direct observation and patient recall of health behavior advice. Prev Med. 2004 Mar;38(3):343–9.
15. Beck KH, Frankel A. A conceptualization of threat communications and protective health behavior. Soc Psychol Q. 1981 Sep;44(3):204–17.
16. Starkman MN, Gebarski SS, Berent S, Schteingart DE. Hippocampal formation volume, memory dysfunction, and cortisol levels in patients with Cushing's syndrome. Biol Psychiatry. 1992 Nov 1;32(9):756–65.
17. Wolkowitz OM, Reus VI, Weingartner H, Thompson K, Breier A, Doran A, Rubinow D, Pickar D. Cognitive effects of corticosteroids. Am J Psychiatry. 1990 Oct;147(10):1297–303.
18. DiMatteo MR, Haskard KB, Williams SL. Health beliefs, disease severity, and patient adherence: a meta-analysis. Med Care. 2007 Jun;45(6):521–8.
19. Croyle RT, Loftus EF, Barger SD, Sun YC, Hart M, Gettig J. How well do people recall risk factor test results? Accuracy and bias among cholesterol screening participants. Health Psychol. 2006 May;25(3):425–32.
20. Gerrard M, Gibbons FX, Benthin AC, Hessling RM. A longitudinal study of the reciprocal nature of risk behaviors and cognitions in adolescents: what you do shapes what you think, and vice versa. Health Psychol. 1996 Sep;15(5):344–54.
21. Festinger, L. A Theory of Cognitive Dissonance. Stanford, CA: Stanford University Press; 1957.
22. Nisbett RE, Ross L. Human Inference. Englewood Cliffs, NJ: Prentice Hall; 1980.
23. Taylor SE, Crocker J. Schematic bases of social information processing. In: Higgins ET, Herman CP, Zanna MP, editors. Hillsdale, NJ: Lawrence Erlbaum; 1981. p. 89–134.
24. Fiske SE, Taylor SE. Social Cognition. 2nd ed. New York: McGraw Hill; 1991.
25. Greenwald AG. The totalitarian ego: Fabrication and revision of personal history. Amer Psychol. 1980;35:603–18.
26. Secchi G, Strepparava MG. The quality of life in cancer patients: a cognitive approach. Eur J Intern Med. 2001 Feb;12(1):35–42.

27. Umberson D. Gender, marital status and the social control of health behavior. Soc Sci Med. 1992 Apr;34(8):907–17.
28. Herlitz A, Nilsson LG, Backman L. Gender differences in episodic memory. Mem Cognit. 1997 Nov;25(6):801–11.
29. Kimura D, Clarke PG. Women's advantage on verbal memory is not restricted to concrete words. Psychol Rep. 2002 Dec;91(3 Pt 2):1137–42.
30. Verhaeghen P, Marcoen A, Goossens L. Facts and fiction about memory aging: a quantitative integration of research findings. Journals of Gerontology: Psychological Sciences. 1993;48:157–71.
31. Spencer WD, Raz N. Differential effects of aging on memory for content and context: a meta-analysis. Psychol Aging. 1995 Dec;10(4):527–39.
32. Harrison Y, Horne JA. Sleep loss and temporal memory. Q J Exp Psychol A. 2000 Feb;53(1):271–9.
33. Maquet P. The Role of Sleep in Learning and Memory. Science. 2001;294:1048–52.
34. Fenn KM, Nusbaum HC, Margoliash D. Consolidation during sleep of perceptual learning of spoken language. Nature. 2003 Oct 9;425(6958):614–6.
35. Peigneux P, Laureys S, Fuchs S, Collette F, Perrin F, Reggers J, Phillips C, Degueldre C, Del Fiore G, Aerts J, Luxen A, Maquet P. Are spatial memories strengthened in the human hippocampus during slow wave sleep? Neuron. 2004 Oct 28;44(3):535–45.
36. Sutherland GR, McNaughton B. Memory trace reactivation in hippocampal and neocortical neuronal ensembles. Curr Opin Neurobiol. 2000 Apr;10(2):180–6.
37. Fishbein W, McGaugh JL, Swarz JR. Retrograde amnesia: electroconvulsive shock effects after termination of rapid eye movement sleep deprivation. Science. 1971 Apr 2;172(978):80–2.
38. Beisecker AE, Beisecker TD. Patient information-seeking behaviors when communicating with doctors. Med Care. 1990 Jan;28(1):19–28.
39. Brug J, Steenhuis I, van Assema P, de Vries H. The impact of a computer-tailored nutrition intervention. Prev Med. 1996 May–Jun;25(3):236–42.
40. Campbell MK, DeVellis BM, Strecher VJ, Ammerman AS, DeVellis RF, Sandler RS. Improving dietary behavior: the effectiveness of tailored messages in primary care settings. Am J Public Health. 1994 May;84(5):783–7.
41. Skinner CS, Strecher VJ, Hospers H. Physicians' recommendations for mammography: do tailored messages make a difference? Am J Public Health. 1994 Jan;84(1):43–9.
42. Petty RE, Cacioppo JT. Attitudes and Persuasion: Classic and Contemporary Approaches. Dubuque, IA: William A. Brown; 1981.
43. Kreuter MW, Holt CL. How do people process health information? applications in an age of individualized communication? Curr Dir Psychol Sci. 2001;10(6):206–9.
44. Holt CL, Clark EM, Kreuter MW, Scharff DP. Does locus of control moderate the effects of tailored health education materials? Health Educ Res. 2000 Aug;15(4):393–403.
45. Kreuter MW, Chheda SG, Bull FC. How does physician advice influence patient behavior? Evidence for a priming effect. Arch Fam Med. 2000 May;9(5):426–33.
46. Swinburn BA, Walter LG, Arroll B, Tilyard MW, Russell DG. The green prescription study: a randomized controlled trial of written exercise advice provided by general practitioners. Am J Public Health. 1998. 88(2):288–91.
47. Laurant M, Reeves D, Hermens R, Braspenning J, Grol R, Sibbald B. Substitution of doctors by nurses in primary care. Cochrane Database Syst Rev. 2005(2):CD001271.

48. Probst JC, Greenhouse DL, Selassie AW. Patient and physician satisfaction with an outpatient care visit. J Fam Pract. 1997 Nov;45(5):418–25.
49. Linzer M, Konrad TR, Douglas J, McMurray JE, Pathman DE, Williams ES, Schwartz MD, Gerrity M, Scheckler W, Bigby JA, Rhodes E. Managed care, time pressure, and physician job satisfaction: results from the physician worklife study. J Gen Intern Med. 2000 Jul;15(7):441–50.
50. Ley P. Memory for medical information. Br J Soc Clin Psychol. 1979 Jun;18(2):245–55.
51. Ley P. Satisfaction, compliance and communication. Br J Clin Psychol. 1982 Nov;21 (Pt 4): 241–54.
52. Jansen J, Butow PN, van Weert JC, van Dulmen S, Devine RJ, Heeren TJ, Bensing JM, Tattersall MH. Does age really matter? recall of information presented to newly referred patients with cancer. J Clin Oncol. 2008 Oct 20.
53. Cassata D. Health communication theory and research: an overview of the communication specialist interface. In: Ruben BD, editor. Communication Yearbook 2. New Brunswick, NJ: Transaction Books. p. 495–503.
54. Bradshaw PW, Ley P, Kincey JA. Recall of medical advice: comprehensibility and specificity. Br J Soc Clin Psychol. 1975 Feb;14(1):55–62.
55. Mathews JJ. The communication process in clinical settings. Soc Sci Med. 1983;17(18):1371–8.
56. Waitzkin H, Cabrera A, Arroyo de Cabrera E, Radlow M, Rodgriguez F. Patient-doctor communication in cross-national perspective. A study in Mexico. Med Care. 1996 Jul;34(7):641–71.
57. Hadlow J, Pitts M. The understanding of common health terms by doctors, nurses and patients. Soc Sci Med. 1991;32(2):193–6.
58. Jackson LD. Information complexity and medical communication: The effects of technical language and amount of information in a medical message. Health Comm. 1992;4:197–210.
59. Phillips D. Medical professional dominance and client dissatisfaction. A study of doctor-patient interaction and reported dissatisfaction with medical care among female patients at four hospitals in Trinidad and Tobago. Soc Sci Med. 1996 May;42(10):1419–25.
60. U.S. Department of Health and Human Services. *Healthy People 2010.* 2nd ed. With Understanding and Improving Health and Objectives for Improving Health. 2 vols. Washington, DC: U.S. Government Printing Office, November 2000.
61. Kalichman SC, Ramachandran B, Catz S. Adherence to combination antiretroviral therapies in HIV patients of low health literacy. J Gen Intern Med. 1999 May;14(5):267–73.
62. Nielsen-Bohlman, L. Health literacy: a prescription to end confusion. Washington, DC: National Academies Press; 2004.
63. Paasche-Orlow MK, Parker RM, Gazmararian JA, Nielsen-Bohlman LT, Rudd RR. The prevalence of limited health literacy. J Gen Intern Med. 2005 Feb;20(2):175–84.
64. Guttman N. Patient-practitioner information exchange as an asymmetrical social encounter: do patients actually know what their practitioners think they know? In: Schement JR, Ruben B, editors. Between Communication and Information. New Brunswick, NJ: Transaction Books; 1993. p. 293–318.
65. Thompson CL, Pledger LM. Doctor-patient communication: is patient knowledge of medical terminology improving? Health Comm. 1993 5: 89–97.

66. Korsch BM, Negrete VF. Doctor-patient communication. Sci Am. 1972 Aug;227(2): 66–74.
67. Samora J, Saunders L, Larson RF. Medical vocabulary knowledge among hospital patients. J Health Hum Behav. 1961;2(2):83–92.
68. Schillinger D, Piette J, Grumbach K, Wang F, Wilson C, Daher C, Leong-Grotz K, Castro C, Bindman AB. Closing the loop: physician communication with diabetic patients who have low health literacy. Arch Intern Med. 2003 Jan 13;163(1):83–90.
69. Seligman HK, Wang FF, Palacios JL, Wilson CC, Daher C, Piette JD, Schillinger D. Physician notification of their diabetes patients' limited health literacy. A randomized, controlled trial. J Gen Intern Med. 2005 Nov;20(11):1001–7.
70. Schwartzberg JG, Cowett A, VanGeest J, Wolf MS. Communication techniques for patients with low health literacy: a survey of physicians, nurses, and pharmacists. Am J Health Behav. 2007 Sep–Oct;31 Suppl 1:S96–104.
71. Villaire M, Mayer G. Chronic illness management and health literacy: an overview. J Med Pract Manage. 2007 Nov–Dec;23(3):177–81.
72. Castro CA. Primacy and recency effects. In: Craighead WE Nemeroff CB, editors. The Corsini Encyclopedia of Psychology and Behavioral Science, 3rd ed. Vol. 3. New York: Wiley. p. 1241–3.
73. Gazmararian JA, Baker DW, Williams MV, Parker RM, Scott TL, Green DC, Fehrenbach SN, Ren J, Koplan JP. Health literacy among Medicare enrollees in a managed care organization. JAMA. 1999 Feb 10;281(6):545–51.
74. International Reading Association, Special Interest Group on Reading and Readability, 1992–1998 report, Newark: Delaware.
75. Glanz K, Rudd J. Readability and content analysis of print cholesterol education materials. Patient Educ Couns. 1990 Oct;16(2):109–18.
76. Morrow GR. How readable are subject consent forms? JAMA. 1980 Jul 4;244(1):56–8.
77. Hochhauser M. Plain language needed. Appl Clin Trials. 2003: 14–5.
78. Houts PS, Doak CC, Doak LG, Loscalzo MJ. The role of pictures in improving health communication: a review of research on attention, comprehension, recall, and adherence. Patient Educ Couns. 2006 May;61(2):173–90.
79. Houts PS, Bachrach R, Witmer JT, Tringali CA, Bucher JA, Localio RA. Using pictographs to enhance recall of spoken medical instructions. Patient Educ Couns. 1998 Oct;35(2):83–8.
80. Moll JM. Doctor-patient communication in rheumatology: studies of visual and verbal perception using educational booklets and other graphic material. Ann Rheum Dis. 1986 Mar;45(3):198–209.
81. Readance JE, Moore DW. A meta-analytic review of the effect of adjunct pictures on reading comprehension. Psychol Sch 1981;18:218–24.
82. Dowse R, Ehlers MS. The evaluation of pharmaceutical pictograms in a low-literate South African population. Patient Educ Couns. 2001 Nov;45(2):87–99.
83. Hosey GM, Freeman WL, Stracqualursi F, Gohdes D. Designing and evaluating diabetes education material for American Indians. Diabetes Educ. 1990 Sep–Oct;16(5):407–14.
84. Levie WH. Research on pictures: a guide to the literature. In: Willows DM, editor. The psychology of illustration, vol. 1. New York: HA, Houghton; 1987. p. 2–50.
85. Fillippatou D, Pumfrey PD. Pictures, titles, reading accuracy and reading comprehension: a research review. Educ Res. 1996;38:259–91.

86. DiMatteo MR, Reiter RC, Gambone JC. Enhancing medication adherence through communication and informed collaborative choice Health Comm. 1994;6(4):253–65.

87. Gambone JC, Reiter RC. Quality improvement in health care. Curr Probl Obstet Gynecol Fertil. 1991;14:151–75.

88. Jordan D. Demonstrating the effectiveness of community based adherence support. Int Conf AIDS. 2000, July 9–14:abstract no. ThPpD1511.

4

Improving Health Through the Development and Management of Habits

---

"Motivation is what gets you started. Habit is what keeps you going".
—Jim Rohn, author and motivational speaker

Joan awakens every morning at 6:30 am; she doesn't even need an alarm. She lies in bed for a few minutes thinking about her plans for the day and listening to her bedside radio, then goes to the kitchen to put a kettle of water on the stove. While the water heats, she takes a quick shower, then enjoys an English muffin and a cup of tea before dressing for work. She carries the same briefcase and drives the same route each day to her office, eats lunch on the same park bench with one or more of a small group of friends. Although the time at which she leaves to return home varies a bit each day, she always listens to her favorite music CDs during the homeward commute. Twice each week she plays racquetball with a friend before cooking her evening meal, and twice each week she enjoys a long walk through her neighborhood after eating dinner. She does household chores, watches television, or chats with friends later on, but after brushing her teeth (and always flossing!) Joan is in bed by 10:30 pm, allowing her eight hours of sleep. She once thought adequate sleep was a luxury and she felt rather proud and diligent when she stayed up late to work on projects or finish reading a book. She has realized, however, that she simply doesn't function as well on less than eight hours of sleep and she now guards this time carefully. She drifts into sleep just as she emerged from it, to the soft sounds of her bedside radio.

Like Joan, each one of us has hundreds, perhaps even thousands, of habits, and many of them are related to our health. "Habit" is often defined simply as one's usual state of being or behavior, regardless of whether it is learned (such as tooth brushing after each meal) or naturally occurring (such as waking up at the same time every day). But in this chapter we will generally use the term "habit" to mean a behavior, or pattern of behaviors, that is purposeful and has been repeated so often

74

as to become automatic or even involuntary. Many of Joan's behaviors are automatic or nearly so. She doesn't have to think about putting the pot on for tea, or how she will drive home. They are not involuntary, though, for if there is a traffic jam on her normal route, she can certainly change her regular path and get home by a different way. Some habits are involuntary, though. If you regularly set your alarm clock to wake you promptly at 6:00 each morning, you might find that even on vacation you still wake up at 6:00 am—despite the fact that you were really looking forward to sleeping in! This demonstrates an involuntary behavior; even if you think to yourself, "I don't need to get up now—I'm going to go back to sleep," chances are good that you will be unable to do so and will eventually just get up.

Habits fall into several categories. Some habits represent variations on physiological necessities. For example, one must eat regularly, yet overeating can contribute to morbidity (e.g., Type II diabetes, coronary heart disease) and eventually mortality. Many people in our society eat huge portions, binge eat, eat far more than the recommended number of calories for their height and weight, or eat mostly foods that are highly processed and nutritionally deficient. Indeed, there are many examples of habitual responses related to food and beverage consumption (both positive and negative). Jack has a bowl of ice cream every night for dessert. Christina drinks two cups of coffee every morning and one each afternoon. Laurie goes through the fast food drive through on her way home from work when she's tired and doesn't want to cook. Marjorie has a salad for lunch every day. Fred mindlessly munches chips while he works on his computer. We can all think of examples of our friends' and loved ones' dietary habits.

A second type of habit involves variations on behaviors that are not required for living the way eating and drinking are, but are nonetheless components of everyday life. These include habitual movement patterns such as having consistently good posture or fidgeting and continually kicking one's leg back and forth when sitting (thus burning more calories than by simply sitting still). These habitual movement patterns may be things that we once worked hard at (such as sitting up straight) or things we do naturally (such as fidgeting), or even things we try to resist (such as nail-biting).

A third type of habit involves conscious decisions about behaviors that are not required for living (but again, may certainly be beneficial), such as going to the gym for spinning classes every Monday, Wednesday, and Friday. Exercise is widely recognized as being beneficial for both physical and mental health, and many people make it a habit to exercise on an almost-daily basis. Yet others would never put forth the effort to make exercise a part of their daily lives. And, although these types of habits may come to feel quite natural with time, they are not likely to become truly automatic or involuntary. You're unlikely to ever be *unaware* that you're attending your spinning class!

Health is not solely determined by behaviors; other factors, such as genetic predispositions and environmental toxins also play a role. But health behaviors are the most prominent *controllable* contributors to health and disease.[1] It is estimated that close to one million deaths occur each year in the United States because of behavioral choices.[2] For example, obesity is associated with the incidence of a number of diseases, including diabetes and high blood pressure,[3] and alcohol overuse has been linked to increased risk of breast cancer.[4]

This chapter focuses on how behavioral habits related to health are formed and maintained over time, and how unhealthy habits can be extinguished.

Forming Habits

The development of a habit, good or bad, is a complex process. Habit formation typically involves both cognitive (thought-based) and neural (biological) processes and requires both repetition of behavior and prompting by things in the environment. Repetition allows behavioral patterns to become encoded in procedural memory, meaning that the behavioral steps can be carried on without conscious thought.[5] This encoding process happens through the actual strengthening of neural connections, the efficiency with which certain neurons communicate with one another, as described in Chapter 3. When Joan first began her job, for example, she relied on the directions she had downloaded from the internet to find her way to the office and then to retrace her path back home. After a few days, however, the pattern of right and left turns had become part of her procedural memory. Now she pays little attention to her route, sometimes finding herself almost inexplicably at home after listening to a Chopin CD. When she recently had to provide driving directions to a work colleague who offered to drop something off at her house, Joan struggled to accurately describe how to get to her house, despite the fact that she drives there from work on a daily basis without even thinking about it. In fact, her "going home" behavior has become so habitual that last week she got in her car after work and began driving home as usual. She had gone several miles before she remembered that she had a dental appointment, even though she'd seen it on her calendar just moments before she left her office. The combination of getting into her car in the familiar parking lot with the late afternoon sun on her back set in motion her normal pattern of behavior despite the fact that her actual schedule that day was different.

Just as patterns of behavior can become habitual, so behaviors and their contexts can become habitually associated; this is what happened to Joan. Through a process called "classical conditioning," environmental triggers are able to exert influence over neural and physiological reactions and these can, in turn, prompt behaviors. It is important to keep in mind that sometimes habits develop effortlessly because their associations or outcomes are naturally pleasant; other habits develop with effort and become more pleasant over time; the latter often characterizes the goals of health behavior change.

Classical Conditioning

Classical conditioning was first described by Ivan Pavlov in 1927 and involves learning to associate unrelated stimuli with one another, so that they become somewhat interchangeable with regard to the outcome they create. Pavlov labeled things that naturally evoke a particular reaction "unconditioned stimuli." Let's take the example of potato chips. In response to a potato chip in the mouth, most people will salivate and this is not a reaction that must be learned. "Neutral stimuli" are those that do not initially create such a reaction (for example, the newspaper will not typically make a person's mouth water). With repeated pairing, however, the unconditioned stimulus can impart some of its power to the neutral stimulus, turning it into a "conditioned stimulus." If one consistently snacks on potato chips when reading the newspaper, opening the newspaper might eventually cause a hungry person's mouth to water!

It is this process that explains one of the facets of habit formation and maintenance. Conscious efforts can be made to create conditioned responses to environmental cues, and these associations, in turn, can foster the strengthening of the habit and preserve it over time. This is because once a habit has been formed, the original goal need not be present in order for the habitual response to be triggered. Other contextual factors might also initiate the behavioral response.[5] For example, Glen has created a playlist of about 20 pop music favorites and he always listens to them when he runs or power-walks. He's started to notice that even simply hearing one of the tunes from someone's car radio prompts him to quicken his steps, and when he hears a coworker humming one of "his tunes" he suddenly feels motivated to take the stairs.

Operant Conditioning

Another way in which habits may be created is through their association with pleasure or reward.[6] Although reward has a physiological component (chemical releases in the pleasure-centers of the brain), the learning process in this case is more cognitive than that seen in classical conditioning because it places more emphasis on the *expectations* for what will follow a behavior. Associating good things (rewards) with performing certain behaviors encourages their repetition, and the memory of past rewards can be prompted by environmental cues, thus encouraging repeat performances of the behavior.[6] In cases where the desired behavior is difficult to achieve, *shaping* can be used to move the person in small steps toward the larger goal. This method also relies on the process of operant conditioning, but instead of rewarding the desired behavior, successive approximations of that behavior are rewarded; when the first step toward the goal has been mastered, it is no longer rewarded and instead the next step must be achieved in order to gain the reward.

Rewards for Behaviors

As we mentioned in Chapter 2, people can be motivated to adopt new behaviors if they have clear expectations for reinforcements (rewards) associated with those actions. Implementing these same rewards has long been recognized as an effective tool for making behavior habitual.[7,8] For example, a person might be able to get him- or herself to walk regularly by indulging in a bubble bath after (and only after) each walk. Effective reinforcement techniques can work very well to help change behavior, but they need to have certain characteristics in order to be helpful. To create a sustainable habit, reinforcements themselves must truly be rewarding to the person. Attention must be paid to what is most desirable to each individual, recognizing that people differently value particular outcomes or rewards. If a person prefers showers to baths and doesn't especially enjoy bubbles, then a bubble bath would not serve as an effective reward. In fact, it might actually deter them from the desired behavior of walking. It is also important to note that the reward should not be something that is counterproductive to the person's health. Rewarding oneself for consistent walking by regularly eating pints of ice cream, for instance, might be great for reinforcing the walking behavior but will ultimately do more harm than good.

Maintaining Habits

It is possible to imagine a pattern of ongoing ideal behavior on the part of a person who has a well-thought-out and consistent system of highly desired rewards for his or her every health-related action. But, perfect reward systems are not exactly realistic. A better goal would be to create behavioral patterns that can be sustained over long periods of time *without* constant targeting and reinforcement.

Reinforcement Schedules

Research is very clear that for initially establishing new patterns of behavior, a continual schedule of reinforcement is most effective; the target behavior should be rewarded every time it is carried out.[9] After a while, partial reinforcement schedules can be instituted; these are schedules in which the desired behavior is rewarded only part of the time. Ultimately, behaviors that are rewarded according to partial schedules are much more resistant to extinction—that is, they will tend to persist for a long time, even in the absence of reward.[10]

Partial reinforcement schedules may be fixed or variable, and may be ratio- or interval-based (see Figure 4.1). Fixed schedules reward a behavior in a fixed fashion—for example, every fifth time a behavior is done. Rewarding every fifth repetition of a behavior represents a *fixed ratio* schedule, since it is dependent on the number of times the behavior occurs. To illustrate, Ethel might keep track of her gym workouts and treat herself to a movie each time she has completed five workouts. Or, she may wear a pedometer and allocate herself an hour of television for every 5,000 steps she takes.

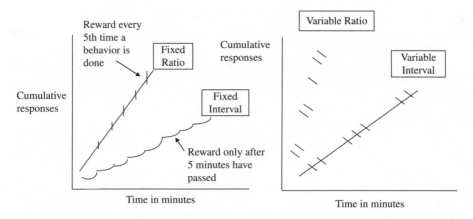

Figure 4.1 Illustration of four types of reinforcement schedules.

A fixed interval schedule could also be based on a time period such as, for example, five minutes. In this case, a behavior can be rewarded only after five minutes have passed engaging in the behavior; then, no more rewards will be attained until five more minutes have passed. Let's take walking on a treadmill as an example. Regardless of how fast or slow Tim walks (and how many steps he takes), he might give himself a point for every five minutes walked. If he's still walking at the end of the first five minutes—one point! At the end of the second five-minute period, another point! If he then walks another four minutes and quits, however, he doesn't get another point (or even half of a point). If Tim has set up a system for himself in which he "buys" rewards for himself with his points, he might be quite motivated to make it just five more minutes . . . and then five more. Depending on what is rewarding to Tim, he might "purchase" weekend time with friends, clothing, tickets to music or sporting events, or desserts (but not too many!).

Variable schedules are just like the fixed-ratio and fixed-interval schedules in terms of the elements of reinforcement except that instead of being "fixed" on a particular number (five repetitions or five minutes) they vary around that number. For example, the reward comes sometimes after four minutes (or 400 steps), sometimes after eleven minutes (or 1,000 steps), and so on. Variable schedules are less predictable and so represent a way of keeping the system of rewards fresh. Higher numbers required for reward might be seen as challenges while lower numbers are unexpected treats. Ethel, instead of simply rewarding herself with a television show for every 10,000 steps might instead make a game of it by rolling dice each morning. She might decide, in this game, that each roll X 100 will give her five minutes of television that evening. If her first roll is $5 + 3 = 8$ then she must walk 800 steps in order to earn that first five minutes of television. If her next roll is "snake eyes" then she will earn the next five minutes of television with only 200 steps. To get a full hour of television, she will roll the dice 12 times and will have to walk somewhere between 2,400 and 14,400 steps. If she ends up on the low end, perhaps she'll decide to roll again and "earn" more TV-watching time!

Implementing these types of schedules alone can be difficult; it is helpful to have someone else to help monitor and regulate the rewards, especially if one is inclined to "cheat" even a little. Utilizing a variety of these behavior modification techniques can also be fun and rewarding as a process! When the process is itself rewarding, positive outcomes and sustainability are more likely. The case study box summarizes Ethel's reinforcement schedule, along with some other examples.

Case Study Box 4.1—Examples of Reinforcement Schedules for Health Behavior Change in Action

Ethel: Ethel wants to increase her walking. She has set up a contingency plan whereby she "earns" her television-watching time each evening in five-minute increments. So that she doesn't get bored with her plan, she has made it into a game. Each morning she rolls dice to see what the "price" of television is for that day. If her first roll is 5 + 5, she multiplies this by 100 and knows that to earn her first five minutes of television she will have to walk 1,000 steps. On her second roll, she might roll a 2 + 4, which gives her 600 steps for her next 5 minutes of television. Depending on which shows are on that evening, she will continue rolling the dice until she has determined how many steps she'll need to take in order to be able to do the television viewing she anticipates. She then keeps track of her steps with a pedometer that she wears from the time she gets dressed in the morning until she goes to bed at night. Ethel allows herself to "bank" extra minutes, and occasionally a show she had earned minutes for isn't as good as she thought it would be. In cases like this, she turns off the television and does something else, saving those minutes for later on. Not only has this strategy gotten her to be more active, it's also made her more discriminating about what she watches on TV!

Mike: Mike is trying to stick to a healthy eating plan, but his office is just down the hall from a vending machine that has a lot of delicious (but very unhealthy) snacks! He found that simply bringing healthy snacks to work with him wasn't enough; he was still succumbing to temptation far too frequently. He has now taken control by creating a barrier to his snack-buying behavior while at the same time reinforcing his healthy eating behavior. He keeps a large, plastic cup in his car and each morning before he goes into the office he puts all of his change into the cup. Since the machine doesn't accept dollar bills, this makes it rather inconvenient for him to make purchases from the machine. The change that he collects in the cup is his "novel money" and it's surprising how quickly it adds up—he counts it each month and it's usually between $25 and $35. He used to feel a bit guilty about spending money on novels (although he loves them, he also thinks they are a bit of a time-waster; and he also knows he could simply borrow them from the library yet for some reason he likes to own them). Now, however, he feels no guilt about buying novels with his change. It's money that would have been "wasted" anyway, and in addition to being wasted, it would have been doing harm to his health.

Continued

The Malley Family: Tim and Denise Malley want their children, Yvonne and Margaret, to learn a variety of good health habits. To help them do this they have instituted a system by which the family saves points in order to "purchase" a variety of activities and other treats. Tim and Denise participate in the system, as well, because they want to model good behaviors for their girls. In the kitchen the family has a rather elaborate chart that lists "point values" for different health-behaviors and a grid on which the family can check off behaviors. For example, here are some of the point values: putting on sunscreen before going outside = 5, tooth-brushing = 5, flossing = 10, drinking a glass of water = 2, eating a serving of fruit or vegetables = 5, washing hands before meals = 5, wearing a helmet when bicycling = 10, putting on a seatbelt in the car without being asked = 2, and so on. Each week the family comes together to add up the points and then the board is erased and the new week of points begins. With their points, the girls can purchase things like media time (watching television or playing on the computer), telephone time, trips to the mall or the park, and so on. These rewards encourage the girls to engage in a broad range of positive health behaviors, with very little nagging from their parents.

Behavioral Contracts and Contingency Plans

In Chapter 2 we introduced the idea of a behavioral contract as a way of motivating patients to make changes in their health behaviors. The idea is that by committing in written form to a course of action, individuals might actually become more motivated to pursue that action, as they endeavor to maintain consistency between their thoughts and behaviors. It is obvious, however, that behavioral contracts can do much more than motivate goal-engagement; these contracts often contain formal schedules for administering reinforcement and punishment and thus can be particularly effective in engaging people to carry out the plan of action they have committed to. Behavioral contracts help to apply subtle social pressure by reminding people that they promised to follow up on the things to which they have made a commitment. Contracts have been found to be effective across a variety of domains from encouraging weight-gain in anorexics[11] to motivating weight loss in overweight patients.[12] In Figure 4.2 a simple contract is presented, but of course some contracts are much more elaborate.

Contingency contracts (also called contingency management techniques) utilize the same principles, typically setting up a system so that target behaviors are readily apparent, providing reinforcements for achieving those behaviors, and withholding incentives when the behaviors are not carried out.[13] Contingency management procedures have also been shown to be effective across a wide variety of clinical settings[14] ranging from self-care for transplant populations[15] to dietary interventions.[16]

Health Behavior Contract

I, _____ Gina Yaakob _____, have decided to set the following health behavior change goal. My goal is _____ Exercise for 30 minutes 5 times a week. _____ I will pursue this goal from _Sept 1_ to Dec 31, 2009. _____ I will do the following to achieve my goal: walking, jogging, yoga class, bicycling, and water aerobics. _____ I will keep a weekly calendar record of my achievements such as the one below

Day of the week	Time	Type of Exercise
Monday		
Tuesday		
Wednesday		
Thursday		
Friday		
Saturday		
Sunday		

If I have been 90% successful with my goal by _____ Dec 31 2009, I will reward myself with _____ a day at the spa, with a massage _____ .

Signature_____ Gina Yaakob _____   Date_____ Aug 31, 2009 _____

Witness _____ Brian Hansen, PA _____   Date_____ 8/31/09 _____

Figure 4.2   Sample behavioral contract.

Some "contracts" may be less formal but still implement some of the same elements as a standard behavioral contract or contingency management contract. They may, for example, come in the form of a worksheet rather than an agreement. By completing the worksheet with their health educator, or perhaps with members in a support group, individuals can solidify their plans for implementing change. Figure 4.3 presents one such sample worksheet modified for use with patients; it is from a format designed to teach health educators.[17] This particular worksheet not only helps patients identify specific actions they can take, and encourages them to commit to these actions, but it also strengthens their self-efficacy by prompting them to call to mind ways in which they have already been successful in changing behavior. This recollection of past successes encourages them to generalize from prior experience to future efforts, enhancing their sense of mastery and competence.

Behavior Change Action Plan

The ONE stubborn behavior I have successfully changed:

Which of the principles we talked about today were used to help change that behavior? (See, you were already an expert in behavior change!)

1.
2.
3.

Which 3 principles you learned today will you commit to implementing in your behavior change plan over the next three months?

1.
2.
3.

For each, explain *specifically* how you will use these principles.

1.
2.
3.

Discuss your action plan with your (health educator / group) and see if they have any advice for you to solidify your plan.

© Tasha R. Howe, Ph.D.
Humboldt State University
Psychology Department

Figure 4.3 Sample behavior change worksheet.

Intrinsic Motivation

Despite their utility, caution is warranted when implementing behavior-modification techniques such as those described in the preceding pages. This is because associating behaviors with external rewards can sometimes diminish the intrinsic motivation associated with those behaviors, as a recent meta-analysis of 128 different studies clearly shows.[18] In other words, people often do better at maintaining behaviors that are supported by their internal motivation/intrinsic rewards than by those that are maintained only to gain an external reward. Part of this has to do with the reward itself. If the reward is instituted to create the behavior but it is not feasible to continue rewarding the behavior over time, then it is likely that the behavior will decrease once the reward stops; the reward was the primary reason for the behavior in the first place. But, if the reward is something that can be maintained indefinitely (such as "earning" television-watching time), then the issue of its possibly decreasing intrinsic motivation is less problematic. The good behavior is likely to be maintained because the reward is available indefinitely.

Verbal feedback is another type of reward that is not only easy to continue over time, but also seems to enhance intrinsic motivation rather than decreasing it.

Examples of supportive verbal feedback are: "You did that really well," and "I'm impressed at how you didn't give up." The effectiveness of verbal feedback is an exception to the general finding that rewards tend to diminish intrinsic motivation. This exception was supported by a meta-analysis which found that recruiting people in a patient's social network to provide positive verbal feedback can serve as an economical and effective strategy for facilitating behavior change. Thus, other people can be valuable helpers in monitoring rewards and keeping individuals from cheating and serve as important influences on a person's willingness to pursue change (as we saw in Chapter 2). In addition, the reactions of other people to an individual's behavior provide potent feedback that can be both rewarding and motivating.

Breaking Bad Habits

We have seen that some habits are easy to maintain over time; they tend to reinforce themselves. For example, eating ice cream every night while watching television can be very reinforcing for some people because it tastes pretty good after a hard day at work. Likewise, for some people, going for a run after work or taking a yoga class can be reinforcing because tight tense muscles finally relax and allow the person to feel less stressed and to relax enough to sleep well.

Unless habitual behavior stops meeting the original goal for which it was adopted, satisfying a goal tends to serve as a positive reinforcement or reward for the behavior, increasing the chances of subsequent repetitions of the behavior. If, for example, you have had several cavities and a painful root canal treatment, you might experience unpleasant anxiety about future oral health problems. But, because you brush and floss your teeth twice a day, you now have healthy teeth and are free of gum disease. You will likely continue this pattern of oral hygiene because you are reinforced for it; having your anxiety about poor oral health diminished makes you feel better. It is rewarding to you. Similarly, someone who works to maintain a healthy weight might feel rewarded each morning when getting dressed, when clothes fit easily and look attractive. The rewards here are looking and feeling good, as well as diminished anxiety over possible weight gain.

So what about those habits that we'd like to extinguish, like smoking, eating high fat fast-food for dinner, and staying up late watching "just 10 more minutes" of our favorite reruns. Why are behaviors sometimes very persistent and hard to get rid of? Why is it difficult, for instance, to quit drinking beer or eating chocolate every day? Partly it is because of the self-reinforcing aspect of many habits that we just described. If we are continuing to engage in behaviors that are not in our best interest, and indeed that may harm us over time, we are not doing so *in order* to hurt ourselves. Therefore, we must be getting some sort of reward for our actions.

The chocolate tastes good and eating it is fun; the beer makes us feel relaxed and drinking it might make meeting new people easier.

In addition, most behaviors are not associated with a single reward. Perhaps the first time you ate a chicken pot pie at age six you really were just hungry. No doubt the pie filled your stomach, thereby achieving the aim, which was to get rid of your hunger. But the pie probably tasted good, too, and since your mother provided it, you may have felt protected and cared for when you ate it. So, while you may be prompted to seek out another chicken pot pie when you are hungry, you might also tend to crave one when you are feeling down or sad or lonely, or simply want to wake up your taste buds. Satisfying one of these latter needs is likely just as rewarding as satisfying your hunger. Once extra associations are learned, new "rewards" become possible—making habitual behaviors much more likely to be reinforced.

So, what is to be done? How can patterns, even those established decades ago, be unlearned? Is it possible to replace our habitual unhealthy actions with fresh, new ways of behaving? Yes, but (no surprise here) it isn't quick or easy. First, to change behavior we need to change what reinforces behavior. The reinforcement systems for unhealthy behaviors will need to be eliminated as completely as possible, or at least weakened, and new competing behaviors instituted to take the place of the old patterns. This process of replacing current rewards with more appropriate ones will take time and many repetitions.

There's no magic number of times that one must repeat a behavior to make it habitual, but the suggestions that are bandied about are never small numbers (like five or ten). This highlights the reality that persistence over time will be required in order to fully install the new "operating system" of health behaviors. What this means in practice is that exercising for a week will likely not be enough to create a habit of exercise, allowing you to let your guard down and naturally continue to exercise. It's also the case, however, that each individual has particular strengths and weaknesses making certain behavioral changes easier than others.

Self-Knowledge and Personality

It's often been said (first by Socrates) that "the unexamined life is not worth living." We might expand this to read, "the unexamined individual is not likely to change." Without understanding one's own strengths, weaknesses, preferences, and tendencies, one is not likely to choose effective strategies for implementing change. Personality refers to a relatively stable set of personal characteristics that are rooted in biological and temperamental factors but have been shaped and molded by the interaction of those factors with the environment. Although it is not the case that personality *determines* people's behavior, it is true that personality influences how we interpret and respond to our environments. (Given our topic, of course, it is especially important to point out that myths about the "nonadherent personality"

Table 4.1 Brief descriptions of the "Big Five" personality traits

Trait	Description
Openness to Experience	Individuals high on this trait tend to be creative and often artistic. They are imaginative and easily in tune with their emotions and feelings. They enjoy playing with and exploring different ideas—they tend to be open-minded.
Conscientiousness	Individuals high on this trait are responsible, organized, and thoughtful. They are competent and orderly, tending to plan things in detail. Their sense of duty is high, and they are generally quite motivated to be successful. These individuals demonstrate a high degree of self-discipline and do not act impulsively.
Extraversion	Individuals high on this trait enjoy being around others—they are friendly, outgoing, and gregarious. They also tend to experience positive emotions and to be generally cheerful. They gravitate toward excitement and their activity levels tend to be high. They are also generally assertive.
Agreeableness	Individuals high on this trait are generally easy to get along with. They are trustworthy and straightforward, connecting with others and understanding their feelings easily. They tend not to be full of themselves. They cooperate well with others, and generally want to make others happy.
Neuroticism	Individuals high on this trait tend to worry. They are anxious and high-strung, can be prone to irritability, hostility, and depression. They also tend to be self-conscious and to feel vulnerable. Impulsiveness is another common characteristic of people high on Neuroticism.
IPIP	The International Personality Item Pool website is designed to allow researchers easy access to measures of individual differences as outlined by the Big Five framework. The actual items (questionnaires) are available along with instructions for administering and scoring the tests, and other general personality-relevant information. No special permissions are needed to use these measurement tools, they are in the public domain. The website address is: http://ipip.ori.org/ipip/

have not been supported by research.) The five fundamental personality traits considered very important by personality psychologists are summarized in Table 4.1.

What does it mean to say that personality is created as a result of interactions between temperament and environment? Let's take, as an example, an infant who is biologically (temperamentally) predisposed to be especially sensitive to the environment, perhaps startling easily and crying heartily. If this infant is raised in a volatile environment where sleeping schedules are unpredictable and parents are inconsistent or unavailable, these biological tendencies may develop into the personality characteristic of neuroticism. An individual high on the dimension of neuroticism tends to worry a lot and feel anxious, emotional, and high strung. That same temperamentally volatile infant, however, if raised in a stable, predictable environment may develop into someone who is lower on neuroticism. He or she may still be emotionally sensitive and attuned to environmental cues, but not overly anxious or moody.

Personality predisposes individuals to interpret the world in particular ways, and makes certain emotional reactions and behavioral responses likely. Therefore, it is not surprising that personality traits are important predictors of many health behaviors. Although personality tends to be stable and unchangeable over time, it does not *determine* behaviors. Understanding one's own personality enables one to use that knowledge to the best advantage.

There is one personality characteristic in particular that tends to be related to adherence and health behavior change, and this is important for a health professional to know about. *Conscientiousness* (the tendency to be responsible, plan ahead, and be organized with good impulse control) is associated with certain better health behaviors including drinking a small amount of alcohol, refraining from smoking, practicing safe sex, eating healthfully, exercising, and adhering to prescribed medication.[19-22] Someone who is high in conscientiousness, however, will also be organized enough to make good use of a daily diary or a chart of the foods eaten or steps walked. For a person low on conscientiousness, regimentation and organization might not be very interesting or motivating at all. Having a requirement of charting behaviors on a daily basis or planning out meals a week in advance is likely to be perceived as tiresome; the person low on conscientiousness may enact the behavior only sporadically or resist it altogether. This person would be better off choosing a different behavioral strategy. The trait of agreeableness is also relevant to health behaviors, with more agreeable people sometimes showing a greater tendency to adhere to medical recommendations and treatment plans.[22,23] Individuals who are more agreeable may be particularly influenced by their perceptions of what their physical therapist, dentist, nutritionist, or other health-care professional wants them to do. They might also respond more readily to suggestions that their behaviors are important to others, such as their children or other family members.

In our example of personality development, we used the trait of neuroticism. An individual's level of neuroticism is also consequential to health behaviors because those who tend to be more anxious are both more likely to notice symptoms of ill health and more likely to worry about what those symptoms mean.[24-26] These tendencies can be channeled to foster positive outcomes, however. In Chapter 2 we discussed what makes a health message persuasive, and you will recall that one persuasive tactic involves invoking fear. A person who is high on neuroticism already has fear and worry, so it might be relatively easy to convince this person of the importance of change. Keep in mind, however, that *overwhelming* fear can be incapacitating, and so a practitioner may need to work with a very anxious patient to actually *diminish* the perceptions of threat. Also, in order for anxiety to be a motivator, the individual must know what she or he can do to minimize the likelihood of the feared outcome.

In Chapter 3 we discussed ways in which messages might be tailored so that patients pay attention to them, understand them, and remember them. These same principles apply when it comes to acting on health-relevant information. Personality is not the sole determinant of behavior, of course. In the last chapter, we noted the particular importance of customizing with regard to health literacy and demographic characteristics. Attending to these factors not only makes understanding and remembering more likely, it also makes change more likely.[27] Knowing about personality and an individual's associated strengths and weaknesses can make it easier to tailor behavior-change strategies so that they complement the individual's natural tendencies. Many questionnaires are available for assessing personality dimensions, but often they are lengthy, costly, or both. In Table 4.1 we provide a link for accessing a Big Five personality assessment tool that may be freely used by anyone wishing to better understand the personalities of her or his patients (or themselves).

Choosing the Right Environments

By the time they reach later adolescence, most people have a good deal of control over where and how they spend their time. A powerful strategy for successful health behavior change involves choosing environments that support the health behaviors we want to achieve. Research shows that when significant others (especially family members) are supportive of good health behaviors, individuals are better able to achieve them.[28,29] Bringing important others into the behavior change plan, then, can enhance the effectiveness of any number of other strategies that might be used. When friends, coworkers, and family members are supportive of our efforts, the environments in which we function for work, play, and family life become extensions of the ideal healthy environment that fosters and promotes health behavior. Seeking out environments where others are engaging in the targeted health behavior is also quite effective—creating a sort of buddy-system![30]

Similarly, spending time in environments where others are engaging in behaviors that we are trying to avoid (e.g., smoking or eating rich, fatty foods) or are avoiding our target behaviors (e.g., failing to exercise) diminishes our chances of achieving behavioral goals.

The physical environment itself can also play an important role in health behavior change. For example, when people have access to exercise equipment or pleasant areas in which to walk safely, they are more likely to exercise.[28,31] People engaging in supervised exercise classes are more active than those "going it alone."[32] Does this mean that in order to effectively carry out an exercise program

Table 4.2 Sample prompts and associated health behaviors.

Prompt	Behavior
Setting dental floss on counter in the bathroom	Flossing
Reminder postcard from dentist's office	Dental cleaning
Shower card with pictures and descriptions	Breast self-exam
Mass media campaign	Seatbelt use
Putting running shoes by the back door	Jogging
Public service announcement	Smoking cessation
Taping pictures of fit people on the refrigerator	Healthy food choices
Putting medication vial next to coffee maker	Taking pills each morning
Drug advertisements	Asking doctor about drugs
Keeping pitcher of filtered water on counter	Increase water intake

one must sign up for classes? Does one have to move to a home in a hilly terrain with beautiful trees and a bubbling brook alongside a walking trail? Of course not! To find a supportive environment, one might seek out nearby parks, low-traffic walking areas, a gym in which to work out alone or with a friend. Or one might look into purchasing some inexpensive exercise equipment to use by the television set when watching a favorite program. Recognizing the availability of opportunities for healthy behavior (such as eating well and exercising) does much to create a supportive environment for actually engaging in healthy behaviors.

Structuring frequent reminders or prompts into one's environment can encourage the use of available opportunities for health behavior.[33–35] Table 4.2 provides some sample prompts, which can help remind individuals about the goals they have set, and encourage them to continue making the decision to pursue their goals. Even when prompted, perhaps the most difficult (but most important) part is *starting* the behavior (e.g., beginning the jog, getting to the gym) because concerns about discomfort, disappointment, or embarrassment can derail healthy intentions. These sources of concern are typically not nearly as bad as people fear, though— especially if people take small steps and "warm up" or "go easy" at first. Thus, simply initiating the behavior is just as important to the overall solution as prompting. After that, other aspects of the context can help to motivate and support the desired behavior. Health-care providers may wish to focus some rewards specifically on taking this first step, understanding that just getting started represents a significant step toward achievement of the larger health-related goal.

Balancing Habits with Mindfulness

When we confront novel situations and consider what actions we need to take toward our goals, we engage in decision making. As we go through the process of making a decision, we rely on our attitudes and beliefs, the prevailing social norms, and our expectations of a likely outcome. We considered these issues in Chapter 1, where we briefly reviewed the theoretical models that explain behavior and behavior change. Here let's consider the example of stress management in order to lower hypertension. As Phil considers whether to try meditation as a way to lower his stress and associated high blood pressure, he remembers a study he heard about recently on the news. The news report described how meditation could indeed be an effective part of a stress-reduction plan. This is appealing to him because he has more faith in trying things that have been scientifically tested, and he also believes that it can be harmful to the body to ingest too many chemicals (so he'd like to avoid antihypertensive drugs if possible). He thinks, too, about his friends and some of the jokes he's heard them make about "new age" things like meditation; in his circle of friends, meditating is *not* the norm. He has to admit that he, too, holds some stereotypes about the kind of person who practices meditation—he doesn't think he fits the pattern. Finally, he considers his own likelihood of success. He anticipates that he might have trouble clearing his mind and doing what is necessary to meditate effectively; he decides that if he does give it a try he will need some help, perhaps a class or two, or maybe a book that describes in more detail how he should proceed.

Phil's decision-making process illustrates how complex even taking on a behavior, much less successfully carrying it out, can be. Much of our everyday behavior, however, occurs in situations that are not novel; it tends to be repetitive and characterized by predictability rather than involving constant decision making.[36–38] We tend to eat, sleep, work, and play in basically the same patterns, whether they are good or bad. We tend to buy the same groceries, drive the same streets, engage in the same hobbies, hang out with the same people, and brush our teeth in the same pattern, day after day. Our habitual behaviors are usually efficient, and take little thought; they are automatic and allow us to focus on other things while we are doing them. The advantage *and* the disadvantage is that they often are "mindless," meaning that they are conducted without a great deal of thought being put into whether or how to do them.[39]

Habits, mindlessly carried out, are great when they embody good health behaviors. They are enacted with little effort and the mind is freed to engage in other tasks. But for automatic behaviors that are not good for health, it is more useful to remove the mindless aspect and instead pursue mind*ful*ness. Consider Ella as an example. Her job as an administrator requires her to juggle many tasks, and one way in which she saves time is by eating at her desk. She has found, however, that when she is "desktop dining" she eats more than she intends to, and although her hunger is sated, she doesn't feel satisfied. She hardly even remembers what she ate, and when she gets home later in the evening, she often feels like enjoying some food, despite the fact that she knows she's not really hungry.

The practice of mindfulness might be effectively employed to help Ella gain control of her eating habits. Mindfulness in eating would involve Ella's slowing down and engaging in the experience of consumption—paying attention to the texture and taste of her food, taking the time to savor it, and focusing on eating as an event rather than doing it alongside some other activity or chore. Studies have shown that mindful eating does tend to decrease the number of calories consumed, as well as fostering a sense of control over one's own eating behaviors.[40-42]

It's easy to see how things that are done regularly become automated and so require less thinking; behaviors that don't require a lot of thought will tend to happen easily and regularly. When behaviors are enacted over and over again, they form a "well-worn path" such that decisions to act, as well as the actions them-selves, flow easily into familiar patterns without the evaluations and decision-making processes that occur before a habit is formed. Evidence of this well-worn path comes from studies of many different health-related behaviors such as exer-cising regularly, practicing safe sex, getting recommended vaccinations, eating and drinking (or not) various foods and beverages, wearing seatbelts, and so on.[36]

But, the effort necessary to create a positive habit (or to extinguish an undesir-able one) will vary according to the complexity of the behavior itself, the character-istics of the person trying to make the change, and the distractions and barriers that present while the change is being implemented.

Managing Barriers to Behavior Change

You will recall that a number of strategies for motivating behavioral change were outlined in Chapter 2. The focus in this chapter has been on implementation of those changes and getting behavioral changes to really stick. Thus far we have empha-sized techniques for initiating and maintaining good habits, but optimizing the formation of good habits also involves understanding the likely barriers so as to forestall their impact. It also requires recognizing the important role that practi-tioners play as they help patients to adopt healthy habits (and get rid of unhealthy ones). Of course, a person must first believe in the importance of making a change and feel competent to do it. This "faith" in one's own competence (self-efficacy) can take time to develop, and by taking on manageable goals, or breaking larger goals into smaller ones, one may come to feel that: "Success is possible—I'm doing it!"

Once these two essential ingredients are in place, though, it is important to be on the lookout for potential saboteurs of one's progress. One common barrier to successful behavior change is an unsupportive social network. Family members who continue to buy and consume junk food when one member is trying to make healthy eating choices or friends at work who smoke (and freely share their cigar-ettes) during breaks present real obstacles for those trying to maintain good health habits.

The monetary costs associated with making health behavior changes can also present a real challenge. Buying workout clothes, organic produce, or prescribed medication may be necessary yet difficult to do if one is on a tight budget. One study found, for example, that after taste—which was most important for determining what participants would eat—cost was second in importance when making food choices; these were followed by nutritional content and convenience.[43] Not surprisingly, cost presented the greatest barrier to low income groups and to younger people (who often have relatively low incomes).

When the targeted health behavior is exercise, physical pain, soreness, or discomfort can be barriers, particularly in the early stages of changing behavior. It is often useful to make sure that people have accurate expectations, so that they will not be surprised and discouraged by muscle soreness or other uncomfortable symptoms. People can also be prepared by encouraging them: *(1)* to notice how these symptoms are decreased, or completely eliminated, over time; and *(2)* to monitor and adjust the behaviors in order to minimize unnecessary discomfort and to make them fit it in with the other demands of their lives, such as work and family.

Limited accessibility is another frequently encountered barrier, whether one is trying to gain access to a clinic, a walking trail, or accurate information about treatment options. Think for a moment about a low-income woman living in an unsafe neighborhood. She works long hours at a desk each day, and rarely gets home before dark. She can't afford to join a gym, and doesn't feel safe walking in her neighborhood after dark. Incorporating physical activity into daily activities is a real challenge for her.

Each of these potential barriers represents a challenge to the person trying to change; being aware of barriers and monitoring one's success in overcoming them is crucial to the process of change.

Self-Monitoring and Regulating

Learning to anticipate problems, cope with setbacks, and keep track of one's own successes and failures all help an individual to constantly improve, and they represent an invaluable set of skills. Through the systems of reinforcement described in this chapter, good health habits can be internalized (that is, the individual can come to take personal responsibility for them and can make them habitual). This is important because, as previously noted, maintaining a system of rewards over a long period of time may be difficult to do. Reaching the final goal and really internalizing the health habits one hopes to achieve, however, can take time. This is why accurate record-keeping and self-monitoring, along with reflection on those observations and subsequent modifications of the plan are so important. Research shows that paying attention to what has been successful in the past, and using these same strategies when implementing new behavior changes can do a great deal to promote success.[30] Without such self-monitoring and strategic adjustments, the road to behavior change will be difficult at best, and perhaps even impossible. Earlier we met Phil, who wanted to use meditation to help reduce his stress levels. In the

Case Study Box 4.2—Phil's Adoption of Meditation for Stress Reduction

Phil was on his way to meet with his health case-manager. At their first meeting, nearly two months ago, they had agreed that he was simply not dealing well with the stress in his life—his job, problems with his stepdaughter, and the strain of his wife's chronic illness were getting to him. They had decided that meditation might be something that would help him manage his stress and control his high blood pressure, as well as being something he might enjoy. Phil felt that despite not seeing himself as a "meditator" he could learn to do it, and he was relieved that this might mean he wouldn't need to start taking antihypertensive medication.

At that first meeting Phil's case manager provided him with some materials explaining some meditational techniques and a DVD to use as he began to practice; they didn't have time to do anything more extensive. Phil was glad to have a plan of action, though, and they agreed to talk again in two weeks.

At their next meeting, they talked about the difficulties Phil was experiencing and worked together to devise a strong, behaviorally based plan to help Phil meditate. Some of the positives that Phil noted to his case manager were that he really enjoyed the soothing music that accompanied the meditation exercises on the DVD. He also noted that the instructions for meditating were very easy; he was surprised, in fact, by how little he actually needed to do! And therein lay one of his problems. Phil was a "do-er" who was constantly thinking, problem-solving, and acting. He reported that he had trouble "clearing my mind" and "letting my thoughts flow like running water the way I'm supposed to." Instead he kept getting distracted by the things he felt he should be doing for work, or by hearing his stepdaughter's conversations with his wife or on the phone with her friends. Phil reported that he had stuck with "the plan" to meditate daily for most of the first week, but had only meditated twice during the week before the second visit with his case manager. He was feeling less optimistic that meditating was something he could do.

The first suggestion Phil's case-manager had for him was to go somewhere else to meditate. He had been closing the door to his study and using the small television and DVD player there, but it was clear that the papers on his desk, and the close proximity to other family members and their conversations, were too distracting to Phil. He needed a quiet place where he could focus on his own thoughts. Together they decided that he might try putting a comfortable chair out in the garage, or perhaps transferring the audio portion of the DVD to a portable device so that he could meditate outside.

The second alteration that they made to Phil's approach was the time frame. Phil had been diligently trying to adhere to the time frame on the DVD—30-minute meditation sessions. Since Phil had not meditated before, and it was quite foreign to him, his case manager suggested that he start with just five minutes twice per day. This would enable him to become familiar with the process without becoming overwhelmed or frustrated by his inability to maintain focus and a clear head for long periods of time. Together they worked out a month-long schedule which would gradually increase the amount of time Phil spent in meditation so that by the end of the month he would be doing full 30-minute sessions. They also worked out a simple system of rewards that Phil could use to reinforce his own progress as he practiced the skill of meditation. He felt that this would be helpful early on, before he really started to notice the more important, reinforcing effects of stress reduction.

> **Continued**
>
> As he walked toward to his appointment today, Phil was again feeling in control and optimistic about his meditation. He realized that it would be a long process, this learning to meditate, but he believed that he could already sense some changes in his reactions to stressful events in his life. He could now meditate for 30 minutes at a stretch, and when intrusions interrupted his concentration he found that he could quickly reorient himself. He had been keeping track of what worked for him and what didn't, and he had a couple of ideas that he was anxious to talk with his case manager about, including tapering off on his reinforcers. He probably didn't need them now, as he was starting to see real benefits from his relaxation and meditation. Phil's case is a good example of how selecting appropriate environments, taking small steps toward a goal, rewarding those steps, and carefully self-monitoring and then adjusting behavior-change strategies can lead to success in the realm of behavior change.

case study box we explore his experience in more detail, as he worked to make meditation a part of his life.

The Health Behavior Internalization Model is a theoretical framework that argues for the importance of both personal needs (such as the needs for self-determination, support, and security) and behavior-related needs (like competence and context) when trying to make new health behaviors part of a person's identity. The process of incorporation or internalization of the new behaviors can itself be motivating, and it can also serve as a mechanism for self-monitoring and maintenance of those behaviors.[44] The most important point here, however, is that the internalization of the new behavior(s) will only happen when the whole complement of factors, both internal and external, is taken into account. Thus, religious beliefs, cultural food preferences, family support systems, peer networks, personality characteristics, job-related stresses and so on must all be integrated into the "plan" for adopting a new health behavior.

Bringing all of these aspects of one's life together to foster behavior change increases the chances for success. For example, in Chapter 2 we discussed how social support, social norms, and social pressures might motivate one to take on the challenge of changing behavior. Adopting a weight-loss goal because you want to be able to run and play with the grandkids (without being too winded), or because you don't want your spouse to be worried about your health, demonstrates the power of these external (social) factors. These same elements (e.g., not wanting to disappoint family members) can be recruited to help one maintain health behaviors, too. Even pets can help us maintain good behaviors. Elizabeth, whose dog Hemi is a four-time national agility finalist, was recently profiled in *Shape* magazine (December, 2008). When she first started agility training with Hemi, she could tell that he had "the speed of a champion" but he wasn't winning because *she* wasn't quick enough. Her desire not to hold her dog back from his potential motivated her toward fitness goals that she hadn't consistently pursued for herself! We, too, find that we are often motivated to take our dogs for walks or jogs. Of course, the physical activity is great for us, too, but we might stay in front of our computers or televisions if not for our canine companions who long for some exercise.

Besides recruiting others to help monitor and direct our behaviors, we must also take on the task of tracking our own progress. Depending on some of the factors discussed earlier, such as conscientiousness or how hectic one's daily schedule is, self-monitoring may be more or less structured. If you have time to write down successes and challenges each day (and if this is an appealing option for you), progress can be monitored in that fashion. Seeing patterns in the challenges and successes you encounter is instructive[30] and viewing personal progress is motivating! If, however, this seems tedious or you feel you do not have time, then imposing this method of self-assessment will likely do more harm than good. In this case, perhaps a few moments in reflection before you go to sleep and quickly jotting down a "+" (successful / easy day), "0" (neutral) or "−" (unsuccessful / challenging day) on a notepad that you keep on your nightstand might be a better way to keep focused and monitor progress. Everyone has good days and bad days, successes and failures. Self-monitoring records make these very easy to see.

Managing Ups and Downs

Is there a trick for maintaining positive momentum through the occasional low points in performance? Fortunately, yes! "Lapses" happen to all of us, and one important factor in determining whether this momentary slip back into bad behavior becomes a more serious "relapse" is how we think about it. Berating oneself about a slip-up and blaming oneself for it tends to be associated with a further continued slide into relapse.[45]

Suppose you are on a diet and attending a party. You've got a set of strategies in mind to help you stay on track (such as eating a protein bar before you leave for the event, using a small plate for your food, choosing mostly raw vegetables to eat, and engaging in conversation far away from the buffet table). But when you arrive you find that the party hostess has made the most wonderful apple pie. It smells so good and everyone is raving about it, so you decide to have just a taste; you end up eating a rather large slice. Now what?

One response is to acknowledge your utter failure at sticking to your diet. You didn't just eat some pie, you ate a whole big slice. You might scold yourself for this behavior, and catastrophize, telling yourself that you've messed up the entire day's worth of healthy eating. Depressed as you are now likely to be, it might be rather easy at this point to write off the ruined day. Since it's a failure anyway, why not stop on your way home and get some donuts and that frosted cereal you've been craving? If it's Friday night, it might be tempting to consider the remainder of the weekend as a disaster and simply resolve to start afresh on Monday. This would enable you to enjoy a pizza, some more pie, and a pint or two of ice cream on Saturday and Sunday. You see the pattern.

Keeping the larger picture (and your generally positive gains) in mind, and thinking about the lapse as a learning experience or a brief error that is easily corrected, makes reinitiating the target behaviors easier. After eating that slice of pie at the party, you might focus on all of the good things you've eaten that week, the exercise you've done, and the fact that you didn't eat *two* slices of pie. Although eating pie wasn't your goal, it was a small slip that can be easily overcome. You might tell yourself that you enjoyed it, you deserved it, and you are now satisfied and motivated to have another good week of eating healthy. You might do a small bit of exercise when you get home, to burn off a few extra calories or increase the duration of your exercise the next day. You might reflect on what you might have done differently—for instance, could you have felt satisfied with a slightly smaller piece of pie? You might seek encouragement from a friend or family member. Responses like this, that don't discourage or focus on the negative, but instead emphasize the overall positive trends and the learning process that the lapse might represent will facilitate a quick resumption of the positive behavior, rather than a

Table 4.3 Lapses and reactions.

Behavioral Lapse	Harmful Reaction	Useful Reaction
Eating a large piece of pie at a party	"I've blown it now. Might as well pig out tonight and start over tomorrow."	"I wish I hadn't eaten quite such a big piece, but at least I didn't lose control entirely. I'm going to walk Toto an extra mile tomorrow and that will help me get back on track."
Losing track of time while having coffee with friends, and missing kickboxing class	"Good grief, I guess this is a couch potato day. Since I'm obviously not exercising today anyway, I wonder if I can make it home in time to see the season opener of that new series . . ."	"Too bad I missed class. I think I'll head over to the gym and see if there is another class I can step in for. If not, I can always do my own workout!"
Last-minute requests from the boss mean missing yoga	"Yoga helps me de-stress so it's too bad I missed it . . . but I think getting some of these other things cleared off my desk might de-stress me, too. I don't care if I'm here until midnight!"	"I could have really used yoga after the stress of this afternoon! I'm going to go home and pull out that yoga DVD that I haven't used in a while; it's a pretty good substitute. Then maybe a nice cup of tea . . ."

Table 4.3 (Continued)

Forgetting to brush teeth before bed (recognizing that it's happened several times already this month)	"I'm already in bed and I'm so tired. It doesn't seem to matter anyway; I've forgotten to brush a bunch of times lately and I don't feel any cavities."	"Oh, glad I remembered! I'm lucky that my teeth are strong enough to withstand the bad care I've been giving them lately. I'm going to be extra diligent to make up for it."
Smoking a cigarette after a period of being smoke-free	"Once a smoker, always a smoker. I knew this whole stopping-smoking thing wasn't very realistic for me."	"One cigarette compared to what I used to smoke is nothing. I'm still making good progress. Let me think about what I was thinking and feeling before I decided to have that smoke. What was different from all the times I've resisted the urge?"
Drinking too much alcohol	"Well, I'm already tipsy—I'm not going to be driving home. And since that's the case, I might as well go all-out!"	"I'm feeling tipsy; if I want to wake up tomorrow without a raging headache I'd better have some water and no more alcohol. Oh, and a multivitamin when I get home, too."

slide into relapse. Some examples of effective (and detrimental) responses to behavioral lapses can be found in Table 4.3.

Recognizing when one is likely to be most vulnerable and taking extra precautions during those times or situations is also a good strategy to employ to avoid health behavior lapses. *Proactive coping* is the term used to describe a strategy in which people actively anticipate potential barriers or problems, garner resources to help deal with them, and maintain vigilance so that when these situations come up they can be dealt with quickly using the resources that have been readied.[46] Resources may be social, personal, or external/concrete in nature, but they must fit the specific challenge. For example, knowing that a party atmosphere will be challenging, you might recruit a friend who will also be at the party to encourage you to make healthy choices and discourage overeating while you're there. A social resource such as this may be more powerful in the party context than a more private monitoring method, such as giving yourself "points" for good food choices. In the party environment it might be easy to say, "Who cares about the points?" and give in to temptation, whereas a social monitor is more difficult to ignore. Depending on how well a particular strategy works, modifications can be made to future plans as part of the proactive coping method. Perhaps you and your buddy can agree that you will go to the gym the day following the party, and that you will do some extra repetitions of exercise or extra minutes on the treadmill if you didn't stick to your eating plan the night before.

The Practitioner's Role

Health-care practitioners are important not only when it comes to complicated health-care issues, complex drug interactions, or immediately life-threatening conditions. Providers represent a powerful force for informing and motivating their patients and assisting them with adopting healthy lifestyle changes. The effectiveness of clinician counseling about health behaviors during medical visits has been demonstrated across a wide variety of domains including diet, exercise, smoking, and alcohol use.[47–54] Clinicians often do not effectively counsel their patients about health behaviors, however. Helping patients to change their habits still occurs at levels far below the ideal.[55–57] Why? Time constraints are one obvious explanation, of course,[58] but that's not the only problem. Clinicians tend to have little confidence that they can manage their patients' behavior change. They often do not believe in the importance of the health behaviors themselves, and sometimes they don't feel that their own role as health-care providers should include helping people to change their behaviors.[59]

Research suggests that the most effective interventions involve many elements, including the behavioral counseling that takes place during the medical visit. Medical visits are appropriate settings for introducing the idea of, and strategies for, health behavior change as well as for helping patients to move along in the behavior change process (see especially the Transtheoretical Model of Change in Chapter 1). Medical visits with various members of the health-care team are also valuable for reinforcing the initial messages provided by physicians or others, but they cannot sufficiently sustain the factors necessary for maintenance. More is needed, such as telephone counseling,[60] video- or computer-based aids,[61,62] personal digital assistants,[63,64] informational leaflets tailored to the patient,[65] and ongoing contact with the health-care team.[66,53] All of these have been found to increase the effectiveness of simple, counseling-style interventions carried out by physicians.

Utilizing these mechanisms can ease time pressures considerably and allow clinicians to more effectively aid patients in finding and reaching important health behavior goals. Video tapes or DVDs can instruct patients in the area of self-care, or can help a patient think through issues, such as by watching others with similar health problems discuss how they dealt with specific challenges or made decisions about their health. Phone calls can be used to motivate patients and to maintain the patient-provider relationship, as well as to remind about appointments. Tutorials, in writing or by phone, can help patients to accurately describe their symptoms or to formulate their questions prior to a medical visit. We will return to examine these various tools in greater detail in Chapter 7, but we mention them here because they are usually under the direct control of the clinician; being aware of them and utilizing them effectively is one of the ways in which the practitioner can fulfill her or his role appropriately.

Cultural Variations

It is clear that people from different cultures respond differently to interventions and what works for one group may not be effective for another.[67,68] When interventions fail, it is often at least partly due to their lack of cultural sensitivity or to features that are not well suited to a particular person or group. For example, instruments may be written in the individual's secondary language, or may advocate approaches that are clearly counter to cultural group norms. In addition, people of different ethnic backgrounds may process information differently because of the interpretations, beliefs, attitudes, and norms that are affected by cultural factors,[69] and they may experience additional barriers to change that are related to cultural norms, such as dietary practices.[70] Some research, for example, has shown that traditional Latino diets include fewer vegetables and more fried foods than would be ideal; thus, implementing dietary changes to increase consumption of green, leafy vegetables (which represent only a small component of many traditional dishes) may present a particular challenge.[71]

Despite these realities, however, studies have reported mixed evidence as to whether interventions must be *specifically* tailored to the patient's culture in order to be effective.[72,73] Being culturally sensitive and taking patients' cultural norms, values, and other characteristics into account during the medical encounter is always a good idea. Getting to know an individual, forming a connection, and establishing rapport are all important components of a robust health-care relationship. Insofar as culture is part of one's identity, it is crucial to attend to it.[74]

Practitioner Expectations

Through the power of expectations and suggestion, practitioners can help patients in developing new healthy habits, extinguishing negative ones, and improving health outcomes. A physician's encouragement, expectation of success, and optimism can all help a patient in the habit formation or extinction process.[75] A physician's confidence can also provide a motivational force for patients that can aid in this process;[76] and positive health outcomes are associated with reassuring and supportive communications expressed by physicians.[77,78] This is known as the *placebo effect*, in which expectations themselves exert influence on perceived outcomes. For example, within the realm of behavior change, if Dr. Winters expresses support and conviction that Ellie can kick her smoking habit, this will undoubtedly lend strength to Ellie's efforts to quit, making her success more likely. Why? The keys lie in some of the concepts we discussed in Chapter 2. First, this stated belief may enhance her self-efficacy. If her smart, well-educated physician believes she can do it, she may be more likely to believe that she truly can. Second, she may be motivated to please her physician, particularly if she and her doctor have a good relationship and rapport, and if she is high on agreeableness. She will likely want to do her best to quit smoking in order to avoid disappointing her physician. Conversely, suggestions (either verbal or nonverbal) that Ellie is likely to fail may in fact set up just such a scenario by lowering her sense of self-efficacy and creating a self-fulfilling prophecy. These "nocebo effects"[79] may be just as powerful as the better-known placebo effects.

Individual Behaviors and Larger Systems

Doesn't the complexity of habit formation and maintenance make consciously changing a habit difficult? Yes, unfortunately it does! Many times our habits are deeply rooted in our early life experiences and fostered by social systems and policies over which we have little direct control. Our early family environments, which are created and sustained by our parents, influence our health beliefs and behaviors in important ways, and although they are certainly not the only contributors, their influence persists at least into early adulthood.[80,81] Direct modeling seems to be the most potent form of influence by parents on their children's health behaviors, but other methods of teaching, such as discussion of health behaviors, can also be effective mechanisms for establishing behavior patterns in children.[82]

Moving beyond the family system, larger societal systems also exert some influence on individual behaviors, although they are not always as effective as one might expect. One primary focus of public health policy is educating and informing the public, thereby increasing the knowledge base and ostensibly improving health literacy. Some of the best-known nutritional educational campaigns in the United States are the *Food Guide Pyramid*,[83,84] *5-A-Day for Better Health*,[85] and the *Nutritional Labeling and Education Act*,[86] which was implemented in 1994. These educational endeavors have seen modest success, with an approximately 10 percent increase in the number of adults meeting the *5-A-Day* goal over a 5-year period and about 66 percent of adults reporting that they read nutritional labels.[34] Data do not strongly link such educational strategies to large-scale societal behavior change, however.[87] This is not surprising, given that these efforts focus on one piece of the Information-Motivation-Strategy model (see Chapter 1): the *information* piece. We have already seen that strategies to move individuals toward action must also involve motivation and a set of effective tools that can be used to implement changes. Governmental policies, however, attend less to factors (such as creating walking trails and bike lanes, or posting signs reminding people to take the stairs to encourage exercise) that have actually demonstrated effectiveness in changing behaviors.[88,89]

Social policies to promote good health and correct harmful habits are also sometimes ineffective because they fail to target specifically enough, or they over-simplify the complex associations between behaviors, other risk factors, and health.[90] Too often they neither address the power of family influences and other preexisting individual differences, nor take into account the patterns of behavior and lifestyle that the person is already pursuing.[91] Health professionals can aid in making information from the larger system more salient to patients—fostering their motivation and helping them to devise specific strategies based on the informa-tion—by integrating what is discussed interpersonally with what patients are hearing from the mass media and other large-scale (such as governmental) educa-tional interventions. By minimizing the dichotomy of messages for the masses versus those tailored for the individual, the effectiveness of each may be enhanced.[92]

Although systemic changes cannot be made by individuals, we can all do things within our own environments and local (personal) systems to promote health. Citizens can vote for environmentally friendly and health-promoting policies. They can talk to their friends and neighbors and encourage them to also make their voices heard, collectively demanding changes that promote good health. Parents can model healthy living for their children (as can teachers and other adults in children's lives), being mindful to not only talk about good health, but to provide living examples of good health-behaviors on a daily basis. Health-care providers can take the time to counsel patients about health behaviors, even if they believe those behaviors to be "commonsense." Each individual has bad habits that should be eliminated, and each of us envisions strengthening healthy beha-vioral patterns. As we call on our social support networks to help us achieve and maintain good health, we can also be supportive of our family members and friends who are trying to make positive changes in their lives. Even if we have had poor habits for many years, we *can* change these habits and replace them with healthy ones. We simply need to begin.

Conclusion

This chapter has focused on strategies for moving from behavioral intention (that is, taking on a behavioral goal) to action. We have reviewed behavioral strategies that health professionals can use to help their patients and that individuals can use to help themselves implement change. We have also discussed ways in which indivi-dual factors such as culture and personality might facilitate or hinder behavioral change and the things that each of us can do to garner support for the changes we wish to make.

In many cases, ideal health behaviors are obvious. On some level we know what we should do, even if we don't fully realize the importance of implementing the change, are not sure exactly how to make the proper modifications, or we know what to do and how to do it, but just can't get motivated. But there are other times when the best choice to make isn't so clear. Data from scientific studies can be difficult for lay persons to interpret or for clinicians to clearly explain to their patients. A patient may be faced with several health issues that influence one another; actions taken to address one will therefore have an effect on the others. In these cases, the ability to clearly evaluate information in order to make the best possible decision is of paramount importance. This is the topic of our next chapter.

References

 1. Koop CE. Physical Activity and Health: A Report of the Surgeon General. Atlanta, GA. U.S. Department of Health and Human Services, Centers for Disease Control and Prevention, National Center for Chronic Disease Prevention and Health Promotion; 1996.
 2. McGinnis JM, Williams-Russo P, Knickman JR. The case for more active policy attention to health promotion. Health Aff (Millwood). 2002 Mar–Apr;21 (2):78–93.
 3. Mokdad AH, Ford ES, Bowman BA, Dietz WH, Vinicor F, Bales VS, Marks JS. Prevalence of obesity, diabetes, and obesity-related health risk factors, 2001. JAMA. 2003 Jan 1;289(1):76–9.
 4. Singletary KW, Gapstur SM. Alcohol and breast cancer: review of epidemiologic and experimental evidence and potential mechanisms. JAMA. 2001 Nov 7;286(17):2143–51.
 5. Wood W, Neal DT. A new look at habits and the habit-goal interface. Psychol Rev. 2007 Oct; 114(4):843–63.
 6. Skinner BF. About Behaviorism. New York: Knopf; 1947.
 7. Dapcich-Miura E, Hovell MF. Contingency management of adherence to a complex medical regimen in an elderly heart patient. Beh Ther. 1979;10:193–201.
 8. Haynes RB, Sackett DL, Gibson ES, Taylor DW, Hackett BC, Roberts RS, Johnson AL. Improvement of medication compliance in uncontrolled hypertension. Lancet. 1976 Jun 12;1(7972):1265–8.
 9. Myers MG, Cowley MA, Munzberg H. Mechanisms of leptin action and leptin resistance. Annu Rev Physiol. 2008;70:537–56.
10. Nevin JA. Behavioral momentum and the partial reinforcement effect. Psychol Bull. 1988;103(1):445–56.
11. Solanto MV, Jacobson MS, Heller L, Golden NH, Hertz S. Rate of weight gain of inpatients with anorexia nervosa under two behavioral contracts. Pediatrics. 1994 Jun;93(6 Pt 1):989–91.
12. Ureda JR. The effect of contract witnessing on motivation and weight loss in a weight control program. Health Educ Q. 1980 Fall;7(3):163–85.

13. Higgins ST, Budney AJ, Bickel WK. Applying behavioral concepts and principles to the treatment of cocaine dependence. Drug Alcohol Depend. 1994 Jan;34(2):87–97.
14. Petry NM. A comprehensive guide to the application of contingency management procedures in clinical settings. Drug Alcohol Depend. 2000 Feb 1;58(1–2):9–25.
15. Cupples SA, Steslow B. Use of behavioral contingency contracting with heart transplant candidates. Prog Transplant. 2001 Jun;11(2):137–44.
16. Cullen KW, Baranowski T, Smith SP. Using goal setting as a strategy for dietary behavior change. J Am Diet Assoc. 2001 May;101(5):562–6.
17. Howe, TR. Behavior Change Action Plan. Arcata, CA: Humboldt State University; 2008.
18. Deci EL, Koestner R, Ryan RM. A meta-analytic review of experiments examining the effects of extrinsic rewards on intrinsic motivation. Psychol Bull. 1999 Nov;125(6):627–68; discussion 692–700.
19. Bogg T, Roberts BW. Conscientiousness and health-related behaviors: a meta-analysis of the leading behavioral contributors to mortality. Psychol Bull. 2004 Nov;130(6):887–919.
20. Christensen AJ, Smith TW. Personality and patient adherence: correlates of the five-factor model in renal dialysis. J Behav Med. 1995 Jun;18(3):305–13.
21. Courneya KS, Hellsten LM. Personality correlates of exercise behavior, motives, barriers and preferences: An application of the five-factor model Personality and Individual Differences. 1998;24(5):625–33.
22. Vollrath ME, Landolt MA, Gnehm HE, Laimbacher J, Sennhauser FH. Child and parental personality are associated with glycaemic control in Type 1 diabetes. Diabet Med. 2007 Sep;24(9):1028–33.
23. Ediger JP, Walker JR, Graff L, Lix L, Clara I, Rawsthorne P, Rogala L, Miller N, McPhail C, Deering K, Bernstein CN. Predictors of medication adherence in inflammatory bowel disease. Am J Gastroenterol. 2007 Jul;102(7):1417–26.
24. Costa PT, Jr., McCrae RR. Personality assessment in psychosomatic medicine. Value of a trait taxonomy. Adv Psychosom Med. 1987;17:71–82.
25. Kolk AM, Hanewald GJ, Schagen S, Gijsbers van Wijk CM. A symptom perception approach to common physical symptoms. Soc Sci Med. 2003 Dec; 57(12):2343–54.
26. Williams PG, Wiebe, DJ. Individual differences in self-assessed health: gender, neuroticism and physical symptom reports Personality and Individual Differences. 2000;28(5):823–35.
27. Rimer BK, Conaway M, Lyna P, Glassman B, Yarnall KS, Lipkus I, Barber LT. The impact of tailored interventions on a community health center population. Patient Educ Couns. 1999 Jun;37(2):125–40.
28. Trost SG, Owen N, Bauman AE, Sallis JF, Brown W. Correlates of adults' participation in physical activity: review and update. Med Sci Sports Exerc. 2002 Dec; 34(12):1996–2001.
29. Zimmerman RS, Connor C. Health promotion in context: the effects of significant others on health behavior change. Health Educ Behav 1989;16(1):57–75.
30. Elder JP, Ayala GX, Harris S. Theories and intervention approaches to health-behavior change in primary care. Am J Prev Med 1999; 17(4): 275–284.
31. Humpel N, Owen N, Leslie E. Environmental factors associated with adults' participation in physical activity: a review. Am J Prev Med. 2002 Apr;22(3):188–99.
32. Ainsworth BE, Youmans CP. Tools for physical activity counseling in medical practice. Obes Res 2002; 10 Suppl 1: 69S–75S.

33. Dolan MS, Weiss LA, Lewis RA, Pietrobelli A, Heo M, Faith MS. "Take the stairs instead of the escalator": effect of environmental prompts on community stair use and implications for a national "Small Steps" campaign. Obes Rev. 2006 Feb;7(1):25–32.

34. French SA, Story M, Jeffery RW. Environmental influences on eating and physical activity. Annu Rev Public Health. 2001;22:309–35.

35. Lombard DN, Lombard TN, Winett RA. Walking to meet health guidelines: the effect of prompting frequency and prompt structure. Health Psychol. 1995 Mar;14(2):164–70.

36. Ouellette JA, Wood W. Habit and intention in everyday life: the multiple processes by which past behavior predicts future behavior. Psychol Bull. 1998;124(1):54–74.

37. Quinn JM, Wood W. Habits across the lifespan. Unpublished manuscript, Duke University; 2005.

38. Townsend DJ, Bever TG. Sentence Comprehension: The Integration of Habits and Rules. Cambridge, MA: MIT Press; 2001.

39. Aarts H, Verplanken B, van Knippenberg A. Predicting behavior from actions in the past: repeated decision making or a matter of habit? J Appl Soc Psychol. 1998;28(15):1355–74.

40. Baer RA, Fischer S, Huss DB. Mindfulness-based cognitive therapy applied to binge eating: a case study. Cognitive and Behavioral Practice. 2005;12:351–8.

41. Kristeller JL, Zumbrun CS, Schilling RF. "I would if I could": how oncologists and oncology nurses address spiritual distress in cancer patients. Psychooncology. 1999 Sep–Oct;8(5):451–8.

42. Kristeller JL, Papps H, Stahl RF. Risk of worsening renal function with nesiritide following cardiac surgery. Am J Health Syst Pharm. 2006 Dec 1;63(23):2351–3.

43. Glanz K, Basil M, Maibach E, Goldberg J, Snyder D. Why Americans eat what they do: taste, nutrition, cost, convenience, and weight control concerns as influences on food consumption. J Am Diet Assoc. 1998 Oct;98(10):1118–26.

44. Bellg AJ. Maintenance of health behavior change in preventive cardiology: internalization and self-regulation of new behaviors. Behav Modif. 2003 Jan;27(1):103–31.

45. Brownell KD, Marlatt GA, Lichtenstein E, Wilson GT. Understanding and preventing relapse. Am Psychol. 1986 Jul;41(7):765–82.

46. Aspinwall LG, Taylor SE. A stitch in time: self-regulation and proactive coping. Psychol Bull. 1997 May;121(3):417–36.

47. Ashenden R, Silagy C, Weller D. A systematic review of the effectiveness of promoting lifestyle change in general practice. Fam Pract. 1997 Apr;14(2):160–76.

48. Brunner E, White I, Thorogood M, Bristow A, Curle D, Marmot M. Can dietary interventions change diet and cardiovascular risk factors? A meta-analysis of randomized controlled trials. Am J Public Health. 1997 Sep;87(9):1415–22.

49. Calfas KJ, Long BJ, Sallis JF, Wooten WJ, Pratt M, Patrick K. A controlled trial of physician counseling to promote the adoption of physical activity. Prev Med. 1996 May–Jun;25(3):225–33.

50. Eaton CB, Menard LM. A systematic review of physical activity promotion in primary care office settings. Br J Sports Med. 1998 Mar;32(1):11–6.

51. Israel Y, Hollander O, Sanchez-Craig M, Booker S, Miller V, Gingrich R, Rankin JG. Screening for problem drinking and counseling by the primary care physician-nurse team. Alcohol Clin Exp Res. 1996 Nov;20(8):1443–50.

52. Marcus AC, Crane LA. A review of cervical cancer screening intervention research: implications for public health programs and future research. Prev Med. 1998 Jan–Feb;27(1):13–31.
53. Mullen PD, Simons-Morton DG, Ramirez G, Frankowski RF, Green LW, Mains DA. A meta-analysis of trials evaluating patient education and counseling for three groups of preventive health behaviors. Patient Educ Couns. 1997 Nov; 32(3):157–73.
54. Wilk AI, Jensen NM, Havighurst TC. Meta-analysis of randomized control trials addressing brief interventions in heavy alcohol drinkers. J Gen Intern Med. 1997 May;12(5):274–83.
55. Ewing GB, Selassie AW, Lopez CH, McCutcheon EP. Self-report of delivery of clinical preventive services by U.S. physicians. Comparing specialty, gender, age, setting of practice, and area of practice. Am J Prev Med. 1999 Jul;17(1):62–72.
56. Lemley KB, O'Grady ET, Rauckhorst L, Russell DD, Small N. Baseline data on the delivery of clinical preventive services provided by nurse practitioners. Nurse Pract. 1994 May;19(5):57–63.
57. Denny CH, Serdula MK, Holtzman D, Nelson DE. Physician advice about smoking and drinking: are U.S. adults being informed? Am J Prev Med. 2003 Jan;24(1):71–4.
58. Yarnall KS, Pollak KI, Ostbye T, Krause KM, Michener JL. Primary care: is there enough time for prevention? Am J Public Health. 2003 Apr;93(4):635–41.
59. Wechsler H, Levine S, Idelson RK, Schor EL, Coakley E. The physician's role in health promotion revisited—a survey of primary care practitioners. N Engl J Med. 1996 Apr 11;334(15):996–8.
60. Fleming MF, Barry KL, Manwell LB, Johnson K, London R. Brief physician advice for problem alcohol drinkers. A randomized controlled trial in community-based primary care practices. JAMA. 1997 Apr 2;277(13):1039–45.
61. Fotheringham MJ, Owies D, Leslie E, Owen N. Interactive health communication in preventive medicine: internet-based strategies in teaching and research. Am J Prev Med. 2000 Aug;19(2):113–20.
62. Marcus BH, Nigg CR, Riebe D, Forsyth LH. Interactive communication strategies: implications for population-based physical-activity promotion. Am J Prev Med. 2000 Aug;19(2):121–6.
63. Stevens VJ, Glasgow RE, Toobert DJ, Karanja N, Smith KS. Randomized trial of a brief dietary intervention to decrease consumption of fat and increase consumption of fruits and vegetables. Am J Health Promot. 2002 Jan–Feb;16(3):129–34.
64. Crawford MA, Harrington TM, Russell TV, Franklin FA, Lorish CD, Turner TJ, Baumann BK. Practice extenders and PDA-based counseling for smoking and unhealthy diet. Ann Fam Med. 2005 Jul–Aug;3 Suppl 2:S41–3.
65. Strayer SM, Rollins LK, Martindale JR. A handheld computer smoking intervention tool and its effects on physician smoking cessation counseling. J Am Board Fam Med. 2006 Jul–Aug;19(4):350–7.
66. Kreuter MW, Strecher VJ, Glassman B. One size does not fit all: the case for tailoring print materials. Ann Behav Med. 1999 Fall;21(4):276–83.
67. Kottke TE, Battista RN, DeFriese GH, Brekke ML. Attributes of successful smoking cessation interventions in medical practice. A meta-analysis of 39 controlled trials. JAMA. 1988 May 20;259(19):2883–9.

68. Fletcher SW, Harris RP, Gonzalez JJ, Degnan D, Lannin DR, Strecher VJ, Pilgrim C, Quade D, Earp JA, Clark RL. Increasing mammography utilization: a controlled study. J Natl Cancer Inst. 1993 Jan 20;85(2):112–20.

69. Guidry JJ, Walker VD. Assessing cultural sensitivity in printed cancer materials. Cancer Pract. 1999 Nov–Dec;7(6):291–6.

70. Perez-Stable EJ, Marin G, Posner SF. Ethnic comparison of attitudes and beliefs about cigarette smoking. J Gen Intern Med. 1998 Mar;13(3):167–74.

71. Otero-Sabogal R, Sabogal F, Perez-Stable EJ, Hiatt RA. Dietary practices, alcohol consumption, and smoking behavior: ethnic, sex, and acculturation differences. J Natl Cancer Inst Monogr. 1995;(18):73–82.

72. Arblaster L, Lambert M, Entwistle V, Forster M, Fullerton D, Sheldon T, Watt I. A systematic review of the effectiveness of health service interventions aimed at reducing inequalities in health. J Health Serv Res Policy. 1996 Apr;1(2):93–103.

73. Orleans CT, Boyd NR, Bingler R, Sutton C, Fairclough D, Heller D, McClatchey M, Ward JA, Graves C, Fleisher L, Baum S. A self-help intervention for African American smokers: tailoring cancer information service counseling for a special population. Prev Med. 1998 Sep–Oct;27(5 Pt 2):S61–70.

74. Carrillo JE, Green AR, Betancourt JR. Cross-cultural primary care: a patient-based approach. Ann Intern Med. 1999 May 18;130(10):829–34.

75. Novack DH. Therapeutic aspects of the clinical encounter. J Gen Intern Med. 1987 Sep–Oct;2(5):346–55.

76. Czajkowski SM, Chesney MA, Smith AW. Adherence and the placebo effect. In: Shumaker SA, Schron EB, Ockene JK, editors. The Handbook of Health Behavior Change. New York: Springer; 1990. p. 515–34.

77. Benson H, Friedman R. Harnessing the power of the placebo effect and renaming it "remembered wellness." Annu Rev Med. 1996;47:193–9.

78. Di Blasi Z, Harkness E, Ernst E, Georgiou A, Kleijnen J. Influence of context effects on health outcomes: a systematic review. Lancet. 2001 Mar 10;357(9258):757–62.

79. Hahn RA. The nocebo phenomenon: concept, evidence, and implications for public health. Prev Med. 1997 Sep–Oct;26(5 Pt 1):607–11.

80. Doherty WJ, Campbell TL. Families and health. Thousand Oaks, CA: Sage Publications; 1988.

81. Lau RR, Quadrel MJ, Hartman KA. Development and change of young adults' preventive health beliefs and behavior: influence from parents and peers. J Health Soc Behav. 1990 Sep;31(3):240–59.

82. Tinsley BJ. Multiple influences on the acquisition and socialization of children's health attitudes and behavior: an integrative review. Child Dev. 1992 Oct; 63(5):1043–69.

83. U.S. Department of Health and Human Services, U.S. Department of Health and Human Services and U.S. Department of Agriculture. Dietary Guidelines for Americans, 2005. 6th Edition, Washington, DC: U.S. Government Printing Office, January 2005.

84. U.S. Department of Agriculture, Center for Nutrition Policy and Promotion. 1996. The Food Guide Pyramid. Home and Garden Bulletin No. 252.

85. Frazao E, editor. America's eating habits: Changes and consequences. Washington, DC: U.S. Department of Agriculture. Information Bulletin AIB-750; 1999.

86. Marcus BH, Owen N, Forsyth LH, Cavill NA, Fridinger F. Physical activity interventions using mass media, print media, and information technology. Am J Prev Med. 1998 Nov;15(4):362, 78.
87. Brownson RC, Baker EA, Housemann RA, Brennan LK, Bacak SJ. Environmental and policy determinants of physical activity in the United States. Am J Public Health. 2001 Dec;91(12):1995–2003.
88. Sallis JF, Bauman A, Pratt M. Environmental and policy interventions to promote physical activity. Am J Prev Med. 1998 Nov; 15(4):379–97.
89. Adler NE, Newman K. Socioeconomic disparities in health: pathways and policies. Health Aff (Millwood). 2002 Mar–Apr; 21(2):60–76.
90. Friedman HS. Healthy life-style across the life-span: the heck with the Surgeon General! In: Suls J, Wallston K, editors. Social Psychological Foundations of Health and Illness. Boston: Blackwell Publishing 2003. p. 3–21.
91. Hornik RC, editor. Public Health Communication. Evidence for Behavior Change. Mahwah, NJ: Lawrence Erlbaum; 2002.
92. Napoli PM. Consumer use of medical information from electronic and paper media: a literature review. In: Rice RE, Katz JE, editors. The Internet and Health Communication. Thousand Oaks, CA: Sage; 2000. p. 79–89.

5

Evaluation of Risks, Decision Making, and Outcomes

Do not put faith in what statistics say until you have carefully considered what they do not say."
—William W. Watt, statistician

Andi is 52 years old, and she has struggled with obesity for most of her adult life. She's tried many different diets, including one where she ate only pickles and lettuce for supper and another where she had nothing but high-energy shakes week after week. While on these diets, she was able to lose weight, but she quickly regained it once she returned to her "normal" eating patterns. Andi also exercises each day (although it is really for only a few minutes, because Andi defines "exercise" generously to include walking from the parking lot to her office at work, and walking one flight of stairs instead of taking the elevator). Feeling hopeless and at times even desperate, Andi is searching for an alternative weight-loss strategy. A friend tells Andi about a new weight-loss pill that promises to "denature those pesky lipids before they can be metabolized by your body." Andi decides to give the pill a try because the testimonials are glowing, and the ingredient list appears to contain nothing but plant extracts. The prospect of not having to count every calorie she eats is appealing; Andi is looking for a quick solution, and this seems to be it.

It is tempting to believe that most people make decisions about lifestyle changes based on well thought-out and carefully reasoned analysis of data and information. We might also tend to believe that most of the information upon which we make health decisions is both accurate and relevant. But a close examination of this issue reveals that accuracy and reason may be far from the process of making health-care choices. The fact is that few people conduct a truly thoughtful and thorough comparison of the evidence, strengths and weaknesses, and benefits and costs, before they try something that promises to improve their lives, and particularly their health. Grocery shoppers are commonly lured by attractive packaging with promises to be "low-fat," or to lower their cholesterol, instead of by the actual nutritional value of some of their food choices. Andi has been lured by the prospect of an easy fix and the fact that, as far as she can tell, nothing harmful appears to be on the ingredient list of her new "wonder drug."

Even when we do make real efforts to be logical in our decision-making, myriad factors enter our decision-making equations, often without our knowledge or attention. In previous chapters, we examined many of these factors in detail (such as our emotional state, cultural background, and the salience of the stimuli we encounter). Although these factors pose many challenges to reasoned decision making, it is also true that a person's ability to make a good decision will be enhanced if he or she can develop a clear understanding of the facts and follow a structured decision-making process in any particular situation.

Does this mean that a good decision *will* be made if one understands the issues and has good data to evaluate? Not necessarily. But without good data, or the appropriate tools with which to evaluate the data, it is not possible to make an optimal decision. Instead, outcomes may be left to chance.

In this chapter we describe and evaluate some strategies for making reasoned decisions based on empirical evidence. We then overview the essential elements that are needed in order to understand health and medical risk information as it is typically presented in medical journals, scientific articles, and news reports, and by manufacturers. We highlight the importance of patients' involvement in making the decisions that affect them, and last we present some tools that can be used in the decision-making process.

Evaluation and Decision-Making Strategies

In some cases, optimal treatments or strategies are clear and decision making is easy. In most cases, however, the evidence is not so clear and some work is required before one can make, and feel confident about, a decision. Even in cases in which studies have explored the efficacy of a particular treatment, it is possible that the study may have been conducted with people who are very different from the individual making the decision; none of the groups of people studied may clearly match the individual. In addition, combinations of treatments that are not currently being considered may have been used, and outcomes different from those of concern may have been measured. These complexities call for a structured approach to organizing the available data.

Medical decision analysis is a formal process for assessing both the probabilities and the importance of various outcomes.[1-3] Medical decision analysis involves several steps including building and modeling a decision tree (a diagram that maps out various possibilities for and consequences for actions, named for the tree-like shape of its branching possibilities). Medical decision analysis also involves obtaining the relevant probabilities, evaluating the tree, conducting sensitivity analyses, and finally using the results to come to a decision.[4] For those interested in learning to conduct such detailed analyses, we suggest some introductory materials and a detailed tutorial, the references for which can be found in Table 5.1. Table 5.2 lists some descriptions and URLs for open-access tools that clinicians can use for calculating risks, estimating treatment-outcome relationships, conducting decision analyses, and carrying out other clinically relevant tasks.

Even without using the full structured approach, however, applying some of the concepts of decision analysis to personal decision-making can result in more thoughtful and reasoned decisions. Understanding probabilities and systematically evaluating many possible actions and outcomes are some elements of medical decision analysis that may, on their own, help the individual to examine possible choices more clearly.

Let us turn to the issue of odds, risks, and probabilities in decision making, as we further examine the process of formulating effective health plans.

Table 5.1 Medical decision analysis information resources and tutorials.

Introductory information on medical decision analysis:
- Richardson WS, Detsky AS. Users' guides to the medical literature. VII. How to use a clinical decision analysis. B. What are the results and will they help me in caring for my patients? Evidence Based Medicine Working Group. JAMA 1995;273:1610–1613.
- Richardson WS, Detsky AS. Users' guides to the medical literature. VII. How to use a clinical decision analysis. A. Are the results of the study valid? Evidence-Based Medicine Working Group. JAMA 1995;273:1292–1295.

Tutorial on medical decision analysis:
- Detsky AS, Naglie G, Krahn MD, et al. Primer on medical decision analysis: Part 1—Getting started. Med Decis Making 1997;17:123–125.
- Detsky AS, Naglie G, Krahn MD, et al. Primer on medical decision analysis: Part 2—Building a tree. Med Decis Making 1997;17:126–135.
- Naglie G, Krahn MD, Naimark D, et al. Primer on medical decision analysis: Part 3—Estimating probabilities and utilities. Med Decis Making 1997;17:136–141.
- Krahn MD, Naglie G, Naimark D, et al. Primer on medical decision analysis: Part 4—Analyzing the model and interpreting the results. Med Decis Making 1997;17:142–151.
- Naimark D, Krahn MD, Naglie G, et al. Primer on medical decision analysis: Part 5—Working with Markov processes. Med Decis Making 1997;17:152–159.

Table 5.2 Resources for clinical calculations.

---

http://www.fammed.ouhsc.edu/robhamm/cdmcalc.htm#Clinic

This website provides numerous calculators including tools for doing decision analysis, calculating disease-test relations, calculating exposure-disease relations, assessing treatment-outcome relations, and other tasks (such as calculating body mass index [BMI]). Calculators can be downloaded for use, free of charge, and tutorials are provided for some of them.

These tools are provided by:
Robert M. Hamm, Ph.D.
Director, Clinical Decision Making Program
Department of Family and Preventive Medicine
University of Oklahoma Health Sciences Center

http://www.mcw.edu/display/router.asp?docid=3131

This website provides calculators for Bayesian analysis, as well as tools for estimating risk for coronary heart disease and determining appropriate LDL cholesterol goals, among others. These tools are primarily for informational purposes and the website cautions that medical decisions should not be made based on these calculations.

These tools are provided by:
Medical College of Wisconsin
Division of General Internal Medicine
(Developed in 1999 by Charles Hu, M.D.; Ron Kneusel, M.D.; and Gary Barnas, M.D.)

http://www.medstudents.com.br/calculat/index2.htm

This website is a resource for many calculations that are useful during the process of clinical decision making though they do not involve the evaluation of risks per se. They include such things as oxygen exchange ratios, mean arterial pressure, cardiac output, and pulmonary vascular resistance among many others. For each calculation, the equation utilized is displayed.

These tools are provided by:
Richard Z. Toptani, M.D.

http://www.palmspot.com/software/Medical/Calculators/

This website provides an extensive listing of medical calculators of all sorts, some of which are useful in clinical decision making (much like the "medstudents" site above) including things like medication dose calculators, and others that would be useful to patients trying to self-monitor and regulate their own behaviors. The latter include things like blood pressure tracking systems, calorie calculators, and fitness monitors. All of these tools can be downloaded; the majority are freeware or shareware. A few are commercial (not free).

These tools are provided by different manufacturers/creators; PalmSpot merely hosts the site.

A Crash Course in Bayesian Methods

At first glance, the phrase *Bayesian Methods* seems a little intimidating! But in reality the concept of a Bayesian approach is simple, and each of us carries out many informal Bayesian analyses in making decisions every day, from deciding how fast to drive on a slick road to deciding just how spicy a dish to order at a favorite Thai restaurant.

Before we examine the Bayesian approach in more detail, however, let us first consider a strict "frequentist" approach that defines probability as the relative frequency of a particular event over a large number of trials or "opportunities" for the event to happen. In science, this is often considered to be a less biased strategy because it restricts analysis to the study under consideration, and discourages both additional information and subjective decisions about which data to take into account from "muddying the waters." Many of the decisions we make every day are based on such probability estimates (e.g., likelihood of rain or snow, traffic conditions, responses of others) and the closer these estimates are to reality, the better the decisions will tend to be. If the meteorologist on your favorite news channel states that there is an 80 percent chance of rain, a decision to carry an umbrella is more likely than if the forecast indicates only a 20 percent chance of rain. Pregnant women frequently undergo screening tests for genetic disorders. If a screening test reveals a 1 in 50 chance that the baby may have a particular disorder, a woman may decide to undergo further testing, whereas if the test reveals only a 1 in 1,000 chance, she may decide that further testing is not warranted.

In contrast to a frequentist approach, a Bayesian approach reflects reality more accurately, because it is more inclusive and constantly updates assumptions and knowledge in a particular area.[5] Thus, the waters may be more "muddy" but this approach reflects the real world more appropriately than simply using a frequentist approach. When deciding whether or not to seek treatment for symptoms, for example, one *might* simply pay attention to the symptoms (a frequentist approach). A person is more likely, however, to pay attention to symptoms and *also* to draw on a larger knowledge base, thinking about past experience with those same symptoms. (For example, they might consider: "When I felt this way before, did I get better or worse? What was my diagnosis? How did I resolve the problem?") This represents a Bayesian approach.

Although many studies in the fields of medicine, public health, and psychology have relied on traditional, frequentist approaches for their statistical analyses, some might argue that Bayesian roots lie at the foundation of their scientific approach,[6] and Bayesian analyses are becoming increasingly popular. Bayesian research methods use an existing knowledge base to set a priori assumptions about what new data will show. Then they test specific hypotheses and use the results of the study to update the knowledge base. This knowledge base is, in turn, used to set the next set of a priori assumptions. The emphasis is on constantly refining and strengthening understanding.

This process is exemplified by the way in which medical devices are tested by their manufacturers, with new models often differing only slightly from the prior devices. Knowledge gained in testing an earlier device is used to make small modifications in the next generation of devices, and then new data are gathered, which can then be used to make further small adjustments. As individuals, we tend to carry out similar "testing" iterations every day, and we rely on our past experiences to guide our future decisions.

Our worldviews and belief systems constitute our "knowledge base," and using this base of understanding we create and test hypotheses about many aspects of our lives including actions taken to improve our health. Suppose that Andi's knowledge base contains the following: (1) pills may help her conquer her weight problem; (2) some pills can be harmful; (3) plant-based derivatives do not fall into the "potentially harmful" category; (4) life will be more fulfilling if only she can reach her goal weight and wear a smaller clothing size. Thus, Andi's working hypothesis is that buying and taking this new pill will improve her life by helping her to lose weight; she purchases the product and begins her own individual experiment to see if it produces the desired effect.

Within the first couple of days, Andi notices a difference—indeed, she's already lost three pounds! But she has also been experiencing diarrhea, lightheadedness, and heart palpitations. After one week on the pills she quits taking them, convinced that they are the cause of her new and unpleasant physical symptoms. Her recent experience is added to her knowledge base, which now includes the fact that plant-based derivatives might indeed be harmful and the potential weight loss benefits do not necessarily outweigh the physical costs.

There are many sophisticated ways in which the Bayesian approach is used. There are specific statistical methods for assessing a priori (prior to experience) probabilities and a posteriori probabilities (those based on experience, like Andi's physical distress). Even without these technical statistical tools, people still make decisions by mapping out the differences between the two, and deciding where the "truth" lies. Note that we have put the word *truth* in quotes because implicit in this approach is the idea that our understanding will change over time as we obtain more and more data. What the Bayesian approach emphasizes for those making decisions about health is the importance of effectively using preexisting information to enlighten interpretations of current information, and then making modifications in our assumptions as the data dictate.

As one example, consider Teresa, who has knee problems, but is fond of speed-walking. In fact, she competes at the amateur level in the sport. Although Teresa experiences pain after longer walks, she enjoys her hobby and is unwilling to stop it. Teresa does stay informed about various holistic methods of pain-relief and she reads about (and tries) different therapeutic shoes. One of her friends suggests newly developed flexible "booties" that can be worn with regular cross-training shoes for additional support. She tries them, but her pain actually seems somewhat worse the first day and much worse at the end of the week. Teresa reads some customer reviews of the booties online and compares what the manufacturer says about foot and knee alignment with her anatomy book from college; she decides to return them and ask for her money back! Teresa didn't use any rigorous techniques to evaluate the data and make her decision, but she did supplement her existing knowledge-base with new information (her own personal experience, reports from others, and information from her college textbook) and then she used this new understanding to decide on a course of action.

As another illustration of the value of a Bayesian approach, consider Anthony's case. As part of his annual physical exam, Anthony had a PSA (prostate-specific antigen) screening which was elevated—a positive cancer test. What is the likelihood that he actually has cancer? That is, despite the positive test result, we still don't know for certain that Anthony has cancer (medical tests are not 100% accurate and the variables they measure are influenced by multiple factors; thus, the base rate for cancer is often less than the validity of the test). And beyond that, if he does have cancer, what should he do about it? Supposing that he does have cancer, there are still numerous options. He may be prescribed a drug to block his body's production of testosterone (which many prostate tumors require for growth); but these drugs have many unpleasant side effects. He might undergo surgery, or radiation therapy, both of which may create problems such as inability to have an erection or problems with bladder or bowel control. He might choose to simply monitor the cancer, getting regular PSA tests to look for change, but only pursuing treatment if these tests show rapid tumor growth. His understanding of base-rate information, and his weighing of the probabilities for various outcomes associated with the treatment options, will all guide his choices in response to his positive PSA test.

As we noted earlier, our preexisting information (or knowledge base) is typically derived from a variety of sources including our culture and past experience. We also sometimes encounter empirical research, although sometimes that research, particularly about health-care products, is conducted or presented by individuals who have a vested interest in the outcome (such as manufacturers of drugs and devices[7]). That information might be distilled through health reporters in the national media who fail to report potential sources of bias[8] or who sensationalize findings to gain and maintain an audience. Garnering an audience is one goal of the media, as evidenced by the fact that prevalence and risk factors for various causes of death are consistently misrepresented. More mundane and common risks such as for heart disease are often minimized and more sensational topics, such as drug abuse and motor vehicle accidents, receive more attention.[9] This mischaracterization of common risks likely contributes to misunderstandings about various health threats. Even when individuals seek out their own information, there is no guarantee that they are getting good information or interpreting it correctly. Recent studies of the types and quality of information available on the internet have been disheartening. One study found that, when evaluated according to the clinical practice guidelines set out by the US Public Health Service, less than 10 percent of websites purporting to promote health behavior change were actually useful.[10] Another study reported that on a variety of common health-related topics, even "credible" websites were only moderately accurate in the information they presented.[11] Our abilities to critically evaluate sources of information and to understand what study results indicate are crucial skills if we are to engage in good decision making.

Let us turn now to an examination of the ways in which risks are presented, and what the numbers mean.

Understanding Risks and Risk Reduction

On October 30, 2008, the *New England Journal of Medicine* reported the findings of two Swedish researchers showing that the risk of a heart attack is significantly increased during the three days following the switch to Daylight Savings Time in spring, and significantly lower on the day after the switch back to standard time in autumn.[12] The reported differences in risk were small, but nonetheless they were statistically significant, meaning that there is little chance that the findings were merely a fluke and not "real." Researchers in medical and public health journals use a variety of specific statistical terms that allow them to communicate with each other about risk. Three terms that are often used are: *odds ratio*, *risk ratio* (or relative risk), and *hazard ratio* (relative hazard). What do these terms indicate and what's the difference between them? Each of these is a relative measure (as opposed to an absolute measure, which is a difference score rather than a ratio) but each presents risks relative to one another in slightly different ways.

Odds Ratios

An odds ratio (commonly abbreviated OR) represents the association between exposure to a particular risk factor and an outcome. It can be thought of as the ratio of odds for experiencing some outcome in a group that is exposed to a risk versus the odds in a group that has not been exposed to the risk. As an example, imagine a group of 100 smokers and a group of 100 nonsmokers. If 50 of the smokers develop lung cancer and 10 of the nonsmokers develop lung cancer, the odds of developing lung cancer for the two groups can be expressed as follows: smokers $\rightarrow$ 50/100 (1:1 odds) and nonsmokers $\rightarrow$ 10/100 (1:9 odds).

The *odds ratio* is expressed as: [odds of lung cancer for the exposed group (smokers) / odds of lung cancer for the unexposed group (nonsmokers)] or [(1/1) / (1/9)] $\rightarrow$ [1/.11] = 9.1. Thus, the odds of getting lung cancer are about nine times greater for a smoker compared to a nonsmoker.

Odds ratios are commonly used in many kinds of studies including clinical trials, case-control studies, meta-analyses, and various forms of survey research. When the outcome frequency is high in the population as a whole (if, for instance, lung cancer naturally occurs in 25 percent of the population) the odds ratio, when it is greater than one, will tend to overestimate the relative probability of the outcome in one group as compared to another. (This relative probability is known as the risk ratio, and it is discussed in the next section). When the odds ratio is less than one (and the outcome frequency in the population is high), the relative probability will be underestimated. Only when a particular outcome happens infrequently does the odds ratio closely approximate the risk ratio. Figure 5.1 illustrates this, showing how risk ratios diverge from odds ratios as incidence in the study population increases.

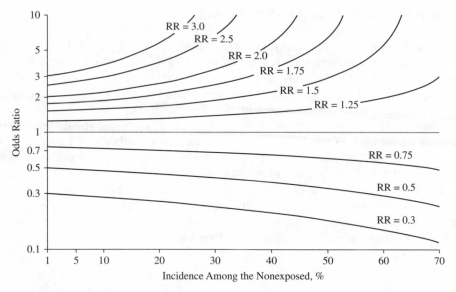

Figure 5.1   The relationship between risk ratio (RR) and odds ratio by incidence of the outcome.

Let's consider, as an example, a real study of neonates using odds ratios.[13] This study looked at disease-related mortality predictors for low birthweight infants in the neonatal units of two separate hospitals. After correcting mortality rates to account for the fact that disease severity was not the same at the two hospitals, the adjusted odds ratio of Hospital One to Hospital Two was 3.27. At first glance, this would suggest that low birthweight neonates in Hospital One had a three times greater risk of death than those in Hospital Two. But in cases like this, where the outcome variable (neonatal death) is common in the study population, the adjusted odds ratio is likely an overestimate of the true risk and it may need to be corrected in order to better represent the actual risk associated with one hospital versus the other.[14] This weakness of the OR approach should be kept in mind when evaluating studies that report their results in terms of ORs.

The same weakness applies whenever a common outcome is being evaluated. Let us say that a clinician is evaluating two summer camps before deciding which he will recommend for his overweight, adolescent patients. He wants them to be successful in achieving their health aims and so he pays careful attention to the OR that describes the odds of reaching the "ideal weight range" during the two-month session (adjusted for starting weight and other factors, of course). He is impressed that, based on the adjusted OR of 2.2 for "Camp Alps" versus "Camp Savanna," the former appears to be clearly superior—more than twice as effective as the latter. He then remembers, however, that reaching "ideal weight range" is common for adolescents attending either camp, so he does a simple calculation to correct for this (referenced in the neonatal study described above) and finds that "Camp Alps" is only slightly better than "Camp Savanna" in helping its campers achieve their weight-loss goals. He decides to let his patients choose which camp they prefer to attend.

Risk Ratios

Just like the odds ratio, the risk ratio (commonly abbreviated RR and also called the relative risk) compares the likelihood of a particular outcome for different groups. As illustrated in the prior section, when the incidence of an outcome in a study population is low, the results from ORs and RRs are almost the same. But the risk ratio contains a slight twist. Here, instead of odds, we are talking about the proportion (or percentage) of individuals experiencing a particular outcome in an exposed versus an unexposed group. So, using our lung cancer example from above, we see that the risk for those in the smoking group is 50 percent, whereas the risk for those in the nonsmoking group is only 10 percent. Our equation now uses these percentages instead of odds: $[50\%/10\%] = 5$. This means that an individual in the smoking group is five times as likely to develop lung cancer as is someone in the nonsmoking group.

This conceptualization is easier to interpret and makes better intuitive sense to most people than does the odds ratio, and so risk ratios are also quite commonly reported in the research literature.[15] It must be noted, however, that some study designs, such as the case-control study, and techniques such as the logistic regression, make it impossible to calculate the risk ratio directly from the data.

We should point out, also, that the interpretation of relative risks can be tricky for a couple of reasons. One is that the RR is dependent on whether we are framing our question in terms of an outcome happening or *failing* to happen (that is, which group is placed in the numerator versus the denominator). Thus, when reading studies that use RRs, we must keep in mind that a small relative change on one side corresponds to a larger relative change on the reciprocal side. Let's use the simple example of gender as a risk factor for Pepper Syndrome (yes, we made that one up). If the male probability of developing Pepper Syndrome is 83% whereas the female probability is only 33%, you will find that your RRs are quite different depending on who is in the numerator. If we divide the male probability by the female probability (.83/.33) the RR is 2.5 but if we divide the female probability by the male probability (.33/.83) the RR is now 0.4. Keeping in mind the fact that 2/5 (0.4) and 5/2 (2.5) are reciprocal fractions will keep these numbers from becoming confusing.

Another reason that interpreting relative risks (or odds ratios, for that matter) may sometimes be perplexing is that the baseline likelihoods are sometimes not taken into account. Consider the challenge for Dr. Sanchez, who enters the examination room to find her usually calm patient, Tyler, agitated. Her queries reveal that he recently read an article that linked a medication he is currently taking with a doubled risk for a rare form of cancer. Although he doesn't have a history of cancer in his family, cancer is salient to him because he recalls vividly the death from cancer of the grandfather of a close friend. Tyler's current medication is serving him well, but after reading this article he doesn't want to take it anymore. He feels he would rather go back to one of the medications he tried before. He prefers dealing with some of their side effects rather than face a twofold increase in his risk for this dreaded disease.

Dr. Sanchez is sympathetic to Tyler's concern; he is absolutely correct in his interpretation of what the study results show. But she points out one thing he has overlooked, which is that the likelihood of this rare cancer in someone with his constellation of characteristics is very low to start with—about one in a million. A doubling of this risk still leaves him with almost no chance of contracting the disease—only two chances in a million. When this additional information is taken into account, Tyler is relieved and glad that he can continue to take his current medications without worry, avoiding the side effects of other medication options.

Hazard Ratios

Hazard ratios (often abbreviated HR or RH for "relative hazard") are a form of what is called "survival analysis"[16] but can practically be thought of as a variation on risk ratios or relative risks. Cox's proportional hazards regression[17] is probably the most commonly used hazard ratio in the health-related literature,[18] and just as with risk ratios, it describes the degree of risk associated with being in one group versus another. One advantage of the hazard approach is that individuals who do not complete the study can still be included in the statistical analysis. These drop-out individuals are said to be "censored," but their data until they dropped out are still valuable.

Survival analyses may, in fact, involve survival—that is, the likelihood of still being alive at a particular point in time. Such analyses might also represent something else entirely, like the "survival" or continuation of a behavior over time. For instance, a survival analysis can be used to estimate an individual's likelihood of continuing to exercise when enrolled in an exercise-support group versus the likelihood when working at exercise maintenance alone.

Whatever the event of interest, the relative hazard represents the probability that it will occur at any given point in time, based on group membership (e.g., a group exposed to a risk versus an unexposed group; a group that received a drug versus a group that received a placebo). Figure 5.2 provides a graphic illustration of relative hazards in the form of survival curves for men versus women. It plots the relative hazard of dropping out of an exercise program according to whether one is exercising alone or with a support group. For both men and women the exercise support group is protective (rh = 0.85)—that is, those who exercise with the support of a group are about 15 percent less likely to drop out than are those who tackle

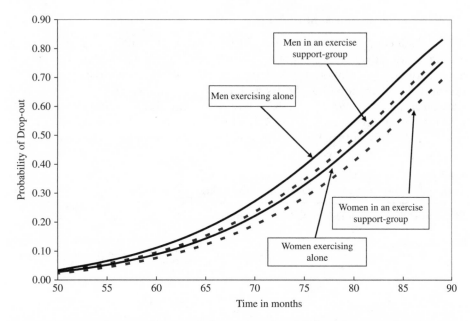

Figure 5.2 Survival curves illustrating the estimated probability of a patient being hospitalized by a given age according to gender and mode of treatment.

it alone. Note that if the question had been framed differently, as the "risk of continuing to exercise" this relative hazard would now be about 1.15, indicating that the likelihood of exercising if you have a support group is about 15 percent higher. The curves also indicate that women are less likely to drop out than are men, so that the individuals most likely to keep exercising (the lowest line on the graph) are women who have an exercise support-group, and those at highest risk for dropout are men who have no support group.

This type of analysis involves a continuous time-hazard function (that is, the likelihood of some event occurring during the next assessment period, if it has not happened already). Therefore, it is describing the relative risk (or protection, if the numerator and denominator are reversed) associated with group membership *at any particular time point.* One common error when interpreting hazard ratios is to assume that they represent relative speed toward the outcome[19] such as looking at an RH for smoking of 1.3 and taking this to mean that smokers die at a 30 percent faster rate than nonsmokers. The correct interpretation is that at any given time point, someone from the smoking group is about 30 percent more likely to be dead compared with someone from the nonsmoking group. If the order of comparison groups is reversed, we see an RH of 0.70, indicating that nonsmokers experience only about 70 percent of the risk of death that smokers experience (at any given point in time).

Straight Versus Standardized Ratios

A final distinction should be made and that is between straight odds or risk ratios and standardized odds or risk ratios. You will recall that in cases where an outcome is common in a population, the odds ratio tends to overestimate risks greater than one and to underestimate those less than one. When the base rate of a condition is very different in two groups, odds or risk ratios can also be quite misleading. An illustration can be found in Table 5.3, which presents two scenarios, each with a relative risk of about two, but with different base rates resulting in divergent results that are misleading if unstandardized.

Table 5.3 Illustration of base rate influences on outcomes.

Scenario 1: Poor outcomes are common (example, hypertension leading to stroke)

	Health Outcome		
	Good	Poor	
Adherent to medications Yes	34	16	50
No	16	34	50
	50	50	100

Standardized Risk Ratio = 34/16 = 2.12
There is slightly more than twice the risk of a poor outcome if patients are nonadherent than if patients are adherent.

Phi Coefficient correlating adherence with health outcome = .36

Scenario 2: Poor outcomes are rare because the disease is very rare

	Health Outcome		
	Good	Poor	
Adherent to medications Yes	49	1	50
No	48	2	50
	97	3	100

Standardized Risk Ratio = 2/1 = 2
Here also there is twice the risk of a poor outcome if patients are nonadherent than if patients are adherent

Phi Coefficient correlating adherence with health
outcome = .058 = .06

In these two scenarios, the actual relationship (correlation measured by the Phi Coefficient) between adherence and outcome is quite different (.36 versus .06) in the two cases even though the risk ratio is almost exactly the same. The reason for this is that the distribution of good/poor outcomes is different. In Scenario 1 the risk of a poor outcome is two times as high with nonadherence and this can be quite consequential because poor outcomes can occur frequently. But a poor outcome, indeed the occurrence of this rare disease, is a low probability event. In Scenario 2, twice the risk is still low.

Thinking About Study Results as a Whole and the Value of Meta-analysis

Each day Peter and Hakim are bombarded with a great deal of health information and advice. Caffeine is harmful to your health . . . coffee can improve your health. Chocolate isn't good for you . . . wait, yes it *is* good for you. Eggs are high in cholesterol and you should eat, at most, one or two per week; wait a minute, eggs contain 22% less cholesterol than previously thought and eating one per day may increase HDL ("good" cholesterol) levels. Confusing, isn't it? Not only are many health messages contradictory but their sheer number is daunting; it's enough to make Peter flop down in exasperation and say, "I give up!" And while this may be a natural approach for many of us, there are others, like Hakim, who embrace each new recommendation enthusiastically. Hakim cuts eggs from his diet almost completely, then adds them back in when a new study shows them to be a healthy part of a balanced nutritional plan; he abstains from all alcohol use until he learns that a glass of wine each day can lower the risk of cardiovascular disease. Margarine, marshmallows, multivitamins, mocha-lattes, and mackerel all appear and disappear from his diet with surprising regularity. By always following the latest health recommendations, Hakim feels assured that, barring an untoward event, he will live a long and healthy life.

   In any given set of research studies, there are usually conflicting results. The odds ratios, risk ratios, and relative hazards described above are very useful when thinking about the likelihoods associated with the outcomes of treatments or health behaviors. But they typically vary from one study to another. No study has all the answers. Studies usually use different methods, and examine different subsets of the many important outcome variables of interest. Each study has its own set of biases, as well, including the method of participant recruitment, the study design, the measurement tools, and the statistical analyses of the data. Because of this, it is possible that even a very well conducted study may miss something important, or may find something that, while true in that sample, doesn't remain relevant in the larger population.

   The way in which study results are presented takes this reality into account. Findings are considered "statistically significant" if they meet some stated (arbitrary, but typical) criterion with regard to their likelihood of having occurred by chance alone. A commonly used cut-off is that of $p < .05$, which means that the probability of being wrong when claiming a finding to be generally true, based on its evidence in a particular study, is less than 5 percent. Another way of saying this is that the likelihood of being right when making such a claim is at least 95 percent.

The statistical term *Type I error* refers to detecting a change (or difference) by chance in a sample when there is not actually one in the population from which the sample was drawn (a false positive). The statistical term *Type II error* involves failing to detect a change (or difference) when it actually does exist (a false negative). As you may already see, these two types of errors are tightly linked to one another. If you adjust your *p* value to decrease the likelihood of missing an effect that really exists, you also increase your chances of "finding" something that merely occurred by chance. Avoiding false findings by setting a more stringent *p* value cut-off also makes it more likely that you might miss something real. Increasing the size of a study sample gives the researcher more "power" to find effects that are real, because as the sample gets larger it more closely approximates the size of the actual population. If there are only 10 people in a sample, it's possible that they happen to be atypical in ways that are important to the study. It is much less likely that a pattern would emerge in a sample of 10,000 if it were not indeed true of the population as a whole.

Studies are not always consistent in their findings because of biases inherent in the way questions are framed, participants are recruited, and data are collected. Inconsistencies also occur because of between-study variations such as sample size and data analytic tools. One way to find out what the "real answer" is (for example, for Hakim to know whether or not eggs really are okay to include in his diet) is to combine the results of several studies. This statistical approach is called "meta-analysis" and it allows researchers to find the areas of consensus among a variety of studies. We have already reviewed the results of several meta-analyses in previous chapters.

A meta-analysis can be thought of as a study in which a number of research studies serve as the "participants." Instead of gathering information from individuals and summarizing it, a meta-analysis pools information from many empirical investigations that all examine the same research question and uses summary statistics to represent the overall results from all studies combined. For example, suppose a meta-analysis examines the question of whether walking reduces the risk of cardiovascular disease (CVD). Indeed such a meta-analysis was done, combining the results from 18 different studies and reporting a hazard ratio for CVD of 0.69 for those who walked the most versus those who walked the least.[20] With a *p* value of less than .001, we can feel confident that walking actually does decrease one's chances of developing cardiovascular disease. The likelihood that the reported findings are merely due to chance and not generally true is less than one in a thousand.

You may be wondering about the studies that were not published because they didn't have significant findings. Studies that don't make it into the scientific literature are not likely to be included in meta-analyses. To address this problem, researchers calculate a number called the "fail safe n," which represents the number of new, unpublished, or not retrieved studies with "no effect" that would need to be included in the meta-analysis in order to make its results nonsignificant.[21] If this number is small, it indicates that the meta-analytic findings are less strong (needing fewer contradictory study results to nullify them). A large number, however, indicates a robust conclusion where many studies would need to contradict the findings before they would be rendered nonsignificant.

If a meta-analysis on a particular topic or research question is available, its results carry more weight than any single study, and results from meta-analyses should be carefully attended to when thinking about implications for various treatment options and other behavioral modifications.

Cumulative and Interactive Effects

You may recall Hakim, who was confused about the many, and often contradictory, health-relevant study findings. His strategy was to adjust his behaviors to match the newest pieces of health advice and to follow as many of them as possible. His behaviors seem to reflect a belief that the effects of these various health behaviors are cumulative. For example, four different studies might suggest four different behaviors each of which can reduce risk for heart attack by 8 percent. If Hakim faithfully carries out each of these four behaviors, can he be assured that his risk for heart attack will be reduced by 32 percent? No, unfortunately he cannot. This is because these behaviors may interact with one another, or "share variance" with one another. That is, taking a pill may reduce his risk, but may then reduce the effectiveness of a dietary change he has also made. Or, the study that found eating nuts to be helpful didn't take into account that those who ate nuts also tended to eat more fruit. Or, the study that advocates eating fruit didn't control for the fact that those who eat more fruit also tended to exercise more. Thus, although each study may be correct, when two behaviors are correlated, adopting both does not yield an additive outcome. And, even if Hakim's risk *was* reduced by 32 percent through some combination of factors, what does that mean? If Hakim's risk was high to start with, a 32-percent decrease is quite important, but if his chance of heart attack was only 15 in 50,000 to start with, a 32-percent decrease in risk doesn't make a lot of difference. Hakim is very young, has low blood pressure, low cholesterol, and no family history of heart disease, so he feels relatively safe that his risk is close to 10 or 15 chances in 50,000.

As we discussed before, a thorough evaluation of options and likely outcomes must include an accurate assessment of the baseline from which one starts. A set percentage decrease in risk is not as meaningful if the risk is very low to start with compared to when the a priori risk is high.

When evaluating study results, it is also crucial to keep in mind the ways in which an individual is similar to, or different from, the sample used in the study. Perhaps the patients in the study were all males and you are female; this may be important in determining whether your risk of disease is the same. And, one must also keep in mind the effects that changing one behavior might have on other risk factors—by either increasing or decreasing them.

Patient Involvement in Decision-Making

The descriptions provided in the section on medical decision analysis focused primarily on the health-care practitioner's role in guiding decisions. But a medical decision should not be a mandate handed down from an authority figure; it should be a course of action that has been evaluated and agreed upon by the patient who will ultimately have to carry out the plan.

An actively involved patient does not imply a passive, uninvolved medical staff; rather it suggests collaboration, teamwork, and shared decision making. The research literature clearly indicates that patients who collaborate in making medical decisions are more adherent to their jointly-decided-upon treatment regimens, more satisfied with the care they receive, and more often experience positive health outcomes than do those who are not involved in treatment decisions.[22–24] Meta-analytic findings indicate that excellent communication (including shared decision making) is related to health outcomes such as patients' emotional health or control of symptoms.[25] In addition, creating partnership with patients is associated with patient satisfaction, as demonstrated in meta-analytic work.[26] In a review of interventions to improve patient involvement and participation in their care, adherence was one of several outcomes that improved as a result of the interventions.[27]

Despite the fact that patients generally want to have a voice in determining the health-care decisions that affect them, it is not the case that all patients are equally well equipped to be participants in their own care. Some patients may not wish to be involved in making health-care decisions at all, and some health-care practitioners are singularly unenthusiastic about engaging patients in the process of making medical decisions.[28] Regardless of the reasons, one study of more than 3,500 clinical decisions made in outpatient facilities found that only 9 percent reflected informed, participative decision making on the part of the patient.[29] Certainly each individual should have the opportunity to be involved in treatment decisions, but research suggests that the way in which (and degree to which) participation occurs will vary from patient to patient.[30–32] Thus, it might be beneficial to ask patients, up front, how much involvement they desire, and to offer them opportunities along the way to be involved in their care.[28] Some simple assessment tools for evaluating preferences for patient involvement may aid this process, assessing things like how much information and discussion a patient would like[33] or even the clinician's preferences for involving patients.[34] Knowing these predispositions ahead of time can smooth the process of collaboration.

It has been suggested that some aspects of the Transtheoretical Model of Change (outlined in Chapter 1) might be used to aid health-care practitioners in working with patients who are at different levels of "readiness" to participate in their care.[24] Different approaches can be used. For individuals who are just getting accustomed to the idea of active patienthood, approaches may differ from those used with patients who have been participants in their own health care for some time.

There are many subtle ways in which physicians and other members of the healthcare team can invite patients to be involved in decisions about their own treatments and health behaviors. These involve soliciting the patient's opinions and concerns, actively listening to the patient's story, and nonverbally communicating sensitivity to and interest in patient preferences. But there are some more formal methods of patient engagement as well, and these are the focus here.

Tools for Participatory Decision Making

Medical decision making requires an individual to make choices about the risks he or she is willing to endure for a particular level of benefit or desirable outcome.[1, 35] For example, one person might be willing to accept a moderate level of treatment-related risk to gain an acceptable but not ideal outcome (e.g., disease management but not cure). Or, given the uncertainties of treatment (such as for menopause or benign prostate conditions), a patient may prefer watchful waiting to any immediate intervention. On the other hand, another person might be willing to accept a very high risk treatment intervention in order to have a chance to attain a very good outcome such as cure. In addition, people vary in the price they are willing to pay in terms of their outcome in order to avoid a highly undesirable condition. Decision trees, one component of clinical decision analysis mentioned early in this chapter, can help patients and members of the health-care team to more objectively and accurately weigh the costs and benefits associated with various treatment options.[2] Given the patient's current condition (including comorbidities—other diseases the patient may have), a set of options is generated. The probabilities of particular outcomes are then listed, and the relative importance or "utility values" are assigned for each.

Let's examine the case of Peter, whom we briefly met earlier in this chapter. Peter tends to give up when he is faced with too many contradictory health behavior recommendations. He has often eaten an unhealthy diet and has gained quite a bit of weight. Partly because of his family history, and partly because of his own habits, Peter has been diagnosed with diabetes. He is in the very early stages of the disease, and has two basic options: *(1)* strict dietary modifications to regulate his blood glucose levels, or *(2)* moderate changes to his diet coupled with drug therapy. The case study box presents a sample decision tree that might be used to help Peter decide how to proceed. This box also presents a quasi–decision tree that illustrates the cost-benefit analysis that Peter might employ, though without the probabilities and utility values found in the actual decision tree.

Case Study Box 5.1—Sample Decision Tree and Simplified Medical Decision Analysis

Peter is facing a decision about how to treat his recent diabetes diagnosis. He still has some flexibility because his disease is in the early stages, and he is considering two options: managing his disease with a strict dietary regimen only (no medications), or taking a more moderate dietary approach and beginning medication now.

The decision tree below shows the two possible results (events) associated with each decision option, and the probabilities for each. The utility (or "value") associated with each outcome is also included. Based on the expected utilities generated by entering the probabilities and utility values, it is more reasonable to take a more moderate dietary approach along with medication at this time (option 2).

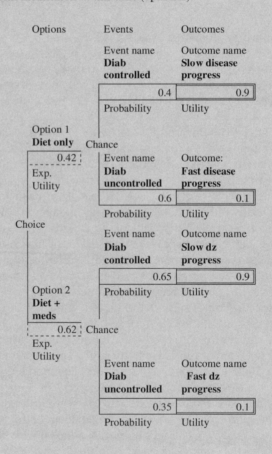

Peter's input here is crucial, because only he knows how important it is to him to eat whatever he wants "for a while longer" versus "practicing self-control" and rarely having his favorite desserts. The decision that must be made represents a "preference sensitive" one, because the ratios of cost to benefit depend, to some degree, upon his personal preferences and values. In this case it is especially important that his health-care provider help him evaluate his options in terms of the scientific evidence.[36] Using a collaborative decision-making process, with appropriate aids as illustrated in the case study box, can result in better understanding of the issues, more realistic expectations about outcomes, less decisional conflict, and a final decision that reflects the patient's values. [36]

There exist a number of methods for engaging patients in risk evaluation and decision making, and many are similar to those discussed in Chapter 3 on informing patients. These methods include interactive computer programs, videos or DVDs that present patients with information about risks, side-effects, and likely outcomes associated with different treatment approaches.[37-39] Sometimes these methods include input from the point of view of patients who have struggled with the same health issues. Others, such as PREPARED®[40, 41] guide patients through various aspects of the decision-making process. For the clinician, web resources provide tools that can be used to guide patients through an informed decision-making process. One particularly useful site is that maintained by the Ottawa Health Research Institute. This website lists numerous topic-specific decision aids, general aids that might be used with any health-relevant decision, a toolkit for health professionals wishing to create their own decision aids, and tutorials to aid clinicians as they develop their decision-support skills. The URL for accessing these tools is: http://www.ohri.ca/decisionaid/. Ideally decision-making aids should be made available to be taken home by patients, so that they can discuss them with their families and friends before a final decision is reached.[24, 42, 43] When used properly, decision aids are beneficial in increasing patients' knowledge and collaboration.[43] Yet, despite the utility of these various tools, individuals ultimately do what they wish, and so a key component of reaching a good decision is patient involvement—no matter how medically appropriate a decision is, if the patient is not involved in making the decision, he or she is less likely to follow through with it.

Conclusion

What makes for a "good decision"? This is not an easy question to answer. A good decision is one that a person feels they can live with, and for which positive and meaningful outcomes are likely. Good decisions cannot be defined purely in terms of the outcome, however, because decisions that have the highest probability of meeting an individual's goals (and thus, are well-reasoned and the best decisions a person could hope to make) do not always lead to positive outcomes. A good medical decision will often help a person to attain a goal that matters to him or her.

Researchers usually measure outcomes like functional status (being able to move and get around and do what one wants to do), quality of life, perceptions of health, symptom reports, and psychological well-being. These outcomes, much like health and illness themselves, are at least partly, and sometimes entirely, subjective. Thus, the answer to the question of what constitutes a "good" decision will depend on the individual patient and situation (see Figure 5.3).

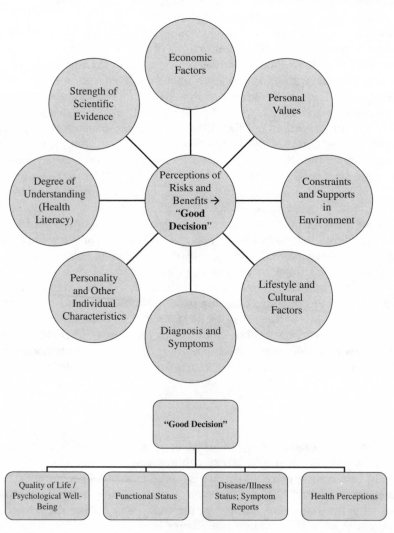

Figure 5.3 Elements comprising the subjective outcome and results of a "good decision".

When, as patients or individuals seeking to change our health behavior, we use the results of research studies to help us make decisions, we must pay attention to many factors, as seen throughout this chapter. For clinicians and patients alike, examining meta-analytic reviews rather than individual studies of a particular research question may give a stronger answer to that question. We must understand the theoretical orientation and methodological limitations of the studies themselves. And, we must recognize that translation from research to application will not be direct; it will be influenced by the individual case of each person to whom we hope to apply the findings. [44]

References

1. Keeney RL. Decision analysis: an overview. Oper Res. 1982 Sep–Oct;30(5):803–38.
2. Speedling EJ, Rose DN. Building an effective doctor-patient relationship: from patient satisfaction to patient participation. Soc Sci Med. 1985;21(2):115–20.
3. Weinstein MC, Fineberg HV. Clinical Decision Analysis. Philadelphia, PA: W.B. Saunders Company; 1980.
4. Detsky AS, Naglie G, Krahn MD, Naimark D, Redelmeier DA. Primer on medical decision analysis: Part 1—Getting started. Med Decis Making. 1997 Apr–Jun;17(2):123–5.
5. Etzioni RD, Kadane JB. Bayesian statistical methods in public health and medicine. Annu Rev Public Health. 1995;16:23–41.
6. Jaynes ET. Probability Theory: The Logic of Science. Cambridge: Cambridge University Press; 2003.
7. Baker CB, Johnsrud MT, Crismon ML, Rosenheck RA, Woods SW. Quantitative analysis of sponsorship bias in economic studies of antidepressants. Br J Psychiatry. 2003 Dec;183:498–506.
8. Hochman M, Hochman S, Bor D, McCormick D. News media coverage of medication research: reporting pharmaceutical company funding and use of generic medication names. JAMA. 2008 Oct 1;300(13):1544–50.
9. Frost K, Frank E, Maibach E. Relative risk in the news media: a quantification of misrepresentation. Am J Public Health. 1997 May;87(5):842–5.
10. Neuhauser L, Kreps G. Rethinking communication in the e-health era. J Health Psychol. 2003;8(1):7–23.
11. Kunst H GD, Latthe PM, Latthe M, Khan KS. Accuracy of information on apparently credible websites: survey of five common health topics. Br Med J. 2002;324:581–2.
12. Janszky I, Ljung R. Shifts to and from daylight saving time and incidence of myocardial infarction. N Engl J Med. 2008 Oct 30;359(18):1966–8.
13. Tarnow-Mordi W, Ogston S, Wilkinson AR, Reid E, Gregory J, Saeed M, Wilkie R. Predicting death from initial disease severity in very low birthweight infants: a method for comparing the performance of neonatal units. BMJ. 1990 Jun 23;300(6740):1611–4.
14. Zhang J, Yu KF. What's the relative risk? A method of correcting the odds ratio in cohort studies of common outcomes. JAMA. 1998 Nov 18;280(19):1690–1.

15. Schechtman E. Odds ratio, relative risk, absolute risk reduction, and the number needed to treat—which of these should we use? Value Health. 2002 Sep–Oct;5(5):431–6.
16. Cantor A. Survival Analysis Techniques for Medical Research. Cary, NC: SAS Publishing; 2003.
17. Cox DR. Regression models and life tables (with discussion). Journal of the Royal Statistical Society Series B. 1972; 34:187–220.
18. Cox DR, Oakes D. Analysis of Survival Data. London: Chapman and Hall; 2001.
19. Tyring SK, Douglas JM, Jr., Corey L, Spruance SL, Esmann J. A randomized, placebo-controlled comparison of oral valacyclovir and acyclovir in immunocompetent patients with recurrent genital herpes infections. The Valaciclovir International Study Group. Arch Dermatol. 1998 Feb;134(2):185–91.
20. Hamer M, Chida Y. Active commuting and cardiovascular risk: a meta-analytic review. Prev Med. 2008 Jan;46(1):9–13.
21. Rosenthal R, Rosnow RL. Essentials of Behavioral Research: Methods and Data Analysis. New York: McGraw-Hill; 1991.
22. DiMatteo MR. Evidence-based strategies to foster adherence and improve patient outcomes. JAAPA. 2004 Nov;17(11):18–21.
23. Golin CE, DiMatteo MR, Gelberg L. The role of patient participation in the doctor visit. Implications for adherence to diabetes care. Diabetes Care. 1996 Oct;19(10):1153–64.
24. Guadagnoli E, Ward P. Patient participation in decision-making. Soc Sci Med. 1998 Aug;47(3):329–39.
25. Stewart MA. Effective physician-patient communication and health outcomes: a review. CMAJ. 1995 May 1;152(9):1423–33.
26. Hall JA, Roter DL, Katz NR. Meta-analysis of correlates of provider behavior in medical encounters. Med Care. 1988 Jul;26(7):657–75.
27. Harrington J, Noble LM, Newman SP. Improving patients' communication with doctors: a systematic review of intervention studies. Patient Educ Couns. 2004 Jan;52(1):7–16.
28. Jahng KH, Martin LR, Golin CE, DiMatteo MR. Preferences for medical collaboration: patient-physician congruence and patient outcomes. Patient Educ Couns. 2005 Jun;57(3):308–14.
29. Braddock CH, 3rd, Edwards KA, Hasenberg NM, Laidley TL, Levinson W. Informed decision making in outpatient practice: time to get back to basics. JAMA. 1999 Dec 22–29;282(24):2313–20.
30. Pierce PF. Deciding on breast cancer treatment: A description of decision behavior. Nursing Research. 1993;42(1):22–8.
31. Rowland JH, Holland JC. Breast cancer. In: Rowland JH, Holland JC, editors. Handbook of Psycho-oncology. New York: Oxford University Press; 1989.
32. Street RL, Jr., Krupat E, Bell RA, Kravitz RL, Haidet P. Beliefs about control in the physician-patient relationship: effect on communication in medical encounters. J Gen Intern Med. 2003 Aug;18(8):609–16.
33. Golin CE, DiMatteo MR, Leake B, Duan N, Gelberg L. A diabetes-specific measure of patient desire to participate in medical decision making. Diabetes Educ. 2001 Nov–Dec;27(6):875–86.
34. Maheux B, Pineault R, Beland F. Factors influencing physicians' orientation toward prevention. Am J Prev Med. 1987 Jan–Feb;3(1):12–8.

35. Barry MJ, Mulley AG, Jr., Fowler FJ, Wennberg JW. Watchful waiting vs immediate transurethral resection for symptomatic prostatism. The importance of patients' preferences. JAMA. 1988 May 27;259(20):3010.
36. O'Connor AM, Legare F, Stacey D. Risk communication in practice: the contribution of decision aids. BMJ. 2003 Sep 27;327(7417):736–40.
37. Kasper JF, Mulley AG, Jr., Wennberg JE. Developing shared decision-making programs to improve the quality of health care. QRB Qual Rev Bull. 1992 Jun;18(6):183–90.
38. Kasper JF, Fowler FJ, Jr. Responding to the challenge. A status report on shared decision-making programs. HMO Pract. 1993 Dec;7(4):176–81.
39. Levine MN, Gafni A, Markham B, MacFarlane D. A bedside decision instrument to elicit a patient's preference concerning adjuvant chemotherapy for breast cancer. Ann Intern Med. 1992 Jul 1;117(1):53–8.
40. DiMatteo MR, Reiter RC, Gambone JC. Enhancing medication adherence through communication and informed collaborative choice. Health Comm. 1994;6(4):253–65.
41. Gambone JC, Reiter RC. Quality improvement in health care. Curr Probl Obstet Gynecol Fertil. 1991;14:151–75.
42. Barry MJ. Health decision aids to facilitate shared decision making in office practice. Ann Intern Med. 2002 Jan 15;136(2):127–35.
43. O'Connor AM, Rostom A, Fiset V, Tetroe J, Entwistle V, Llewellyn-Thomas H, Holmes-Rovner M, Barry M, Jones J. Decision aids for patients facing health treatment or screening decisions: systematic review. BMJ. 1999 Sep 18;319(7212):731–4.
44. Patrick DL, Chiang YP. Measurement of health outcomes in treatment effectiveness evaluations: conceptual and methodological challenges. Med Care. 2000 Sep;38(9 Suppl):II14–25.

6

Relationships and Communication Between Caregivers and Patients

Listening well is as powerful a means of communication and influence as to talk well.
—John Marshall, former Chief Justice, U.S. Supreme Court

Dr. Brenton cheerily greets his longtime patient. "It's good to see you, Sylvia," he says, "How have things been since I saw you three months ago?" After a quick glance at the chart, Dr. Brenton leans against the examining table where Sylvia sits and meets her gaze before asking, "Do you think we made the right decision in switching your pain meds? Have your side effects gone away?" Sylvia launches into her reply, conversing easily with her physician. She feels cared for, empowered, and comfortable being honest about her experiences with her treatment plan. Sylvia believes that Dr. Brenton is concerned for her health and well-being, and that her opinions and perceptions about her own health matter a great deal. She likes that Dr. Brenton doesn't shy away from difficult topics, such as the challenge of managing her chronic pain, and he doesn't treat her like she's abnormal or imagining her symptoms. She views Dr. Brenton not only as a good physician but also as her friend.

After finishing his visit with Sylvia, Dr. Brenton goes down the hall to the examining room where Alvin waits. Just as before, Dr. Brenton's greeting is friendly and almost immediately he asks Alvin for input about his heartburn and accompanying symptoms. Dr. Brenton sincerely wants to know whether Alvin thinks medication or lifestyle change is the best possible strategy for managing them. Dr. Brenton stands close to Alvin and maintains eye contact, indicating active listening and true interest in what Alvin is saying. But unlike Sylvia, Alvin feels uncomfortable with what he considers to be Dr. Brenton's violation of his personal space. He also wonders why Dr. Brenton is asking for his opinion; after all, *he* doesn't have a medical degree—that's why he's here!

In this example, the physician's behavior is consistent over time. He demonstrates an active concern for his patients and makes an effort to collaborate with them in the process of their medical care. Yet these two patients react quite differently to what Dr. Brenton probably views as an "ideal" interactional style. Patients differ in their preferences for health care and for the behavior of their health-care providers.[1-3] This is important to recognize because, as we have noted before, health behavior change and treatment adherence can be heavily influenced by the context in which health messages and recommendations for behaviors are communicated. As we noted in Chapter 5, active involvement in decision making is an important part of this process, but this evaluative process also takes place within the context of a relationship. Several basic models of the patient-practitioner relationship have been identified by theorists and researchers, and we will first briefly outline three of these as they are commonly used and understood. Then, we will spend some time discussing various elements of communication as they pertain to practitioners and patients and how communication processes influence patient adherence and health behavior change.

Models of Practitioner-Patient Relationships

Many labels have been applied to the ways in which patients and their health-care providers interact; these labels often explain how power, control, and decision making are shared (or not) in the relationship. Although the labels may vary and the underlying concepts differ somewhat, there are four commonly encountered categorical distinctions that represent types of practitioner-patient relationships. These are: *paternalism, expertise, consumerism,* and *mutuality.*

Paternalism

A "paternalistic" relationship is one in which the patient is relatively acquiescent and unassertive, providing information when asked and following instructions without much question or discussion.[4, 5] Paternalism is viewed as similar to the relationship between a parent and child,[6] with one party (health-care professional) holding most of the status, decision-making power, and information, and the other party (patient) following along, guided by the directives of the medical expert. This framework views the health-care provider as trustworthy and beneficent, and as using the best medical practices possible because she or he cares for the patient as would a loving parent; correspondingly, it permits the medical professional to compel obedience, as parents also frequently do. Consider the following excerpt from the original Hippocratic Law, which illustrates the paternalistic model: "the physician must not only be prepared to do what is right himself, but also to make the patient, the attendants, and the externals cooperate."

Of course, such an approach casts patient concerns or differing opinions in a less-than-positive light.[7] Prior to the 1980s, a paternalistic relationship between physician and patient occurred more commonly than any other,[8] but some have argued that paternalism fosters an unhealthy level of dependency on the part of the patient. Such dependency may counter the patient's true best interests.[9] And, although some patients do at times prefer a paternalistic approach, especially when they are quite ill,[10, 11] a "consumerist" style has grown in popularity over the past decades,[5, 12] especially as the provision of health care in the United States has changed.

Expertise

The "expert" model of the physician-patient relationship falls between the paternalistic and the consumerist styles. It emerged when medicine became more professionalized in the 1920s, and while it shared the paternalistic model's emphasis on the principles of beneficence, fidelity, nonmalfeasance, and confidentiality, this model was based less on guardianship (which was foundational in the paternalistic model) and more on professional competence. As a result, it became less expected of physicians to make personal (particularly financial) sacrifices for patients, and in turn, patients were increasingly expected to make decisions about their care, setting the stage for the consumer model that characterizes much of modern health care.

Consumerism

A consumerist view of patienthood rose out of a more general concern over protecting individuals from overzealous providers of medical products and services.[13] As such, consumerism views patients as purchasers of a product (i.e., their health care) with an overriding philosophy of *caveat emptor* (buyer beware). This approach emphasizes the rights of patients as consumers of medical information and medical care, and highlights accountability on the part of those who provide that information and care.[7] In 1991 the Patient Self-Determination Act mandated, among other things, that patients must be made aware of their rights to participate in making medical decisions and this law did much to formalize the elements of a consumerist approach. In a consumerist relationship the patient holds a good deal of power because decisions to continue or discontinue care lie with the patient as the purchaser of that care. Thus, a consumerist encounter is ideally characterized by questions and directions from the patient, and by information provided by the patient to the provider.[14] Most recently, the consumer approach has been given further impetus by the availability, to patients, of massive amounts of medical information on the internet and by direct-to-consumer advertising from pharmaceutical companies.

Mutuality

A third type of patient-practitioner relationship is one of mutual participation and collaboration, often referred to as "mutuality."[5] Here, both patient and health-care provider are viewed as experts; the patient is an expert about his or her symptoms, medical history, lifestyle, and preferences; and the physician or other health

Table 6.1 Repertoire of doctor-patient relationships and their appropriate contexts.[19]

Role of Physician	Goal of Physician	Example Context
Expert-in-Charge	Make decisions and carry them out	Emergency situation (e.g., heart attack)
Expert-Guide	Give the patient information, make recommendations, and provide treatment	Less serious situations such as lacerations (e.g., fishhook lodged in eyebrow)
Partner	Build a partnership with the patient; motivate the patient to follow treatment, provide information, and guide decision making	Chronic illnesses (e.g., diabetes)
Facilitator	Facilitate for and motivate patients, often following their lead	Well-controlled chronic illness (e.g., asthma)

professional is an expert about medical matters. With mutual participation, power is shared between the two parties as they work together to make decisions that will result in the best possible outcomes for the patient.[15] In this type of relationship, an active exchange of ideas and open negotiation of differences results in power-sharing and the patient's ability to make personal health-care decisions, taking into account his or her needs and abilities while also being fully informed by the medical knowledge and experience of the medical expert.[16, 17] The mutuality model relies heavily on each member of the health-care partnership but is nonetheless patient-centered.[18] The relationship is mutual in its *focus* because the patient's best interest is paramount, and in its *effort* because both parties are fully engaged in the patient's care. Table 6.1 summarizes situational contexts in which different models of physician-patient relationships might be most appropriate; these have been adapted from a commentary by Lussier and Richard[19] in which it can be seen that the "expert-in-charge" approach is analogous to the "paternalistic" model discussed above; the "partner" approach reflects this chapter's model of "mutuality"; the "facilitator" approach is similar though not equivalent to the "consumerist" model presented here; and the "expert-guide" approach falls some-where between paternalism and partnership.

Practitioner-Patient Communication

Within the context of the practitioner-patient relationship, communication comprises both a primary task and a useful tool.[20-22] As early as 1899, Sir William Osler taught that patients would reveal the diagnosis to their physicians, if only the physicians would listen. Today, some would argue that communication is the most important ingredient in medical care,[5] and both the *American College of Graduate*

Medical Education (www.acgme.org) and the *Association of American Medical Colleges* (www.aamc.org) recognize the crucial role that communication plays by requiring competency in interpersonal communication as a core skill in medical practice. Despite its importance, and the vast body of research that exists on the topic, the communication that takes place between patients and their health-care providers tends to take on unique characteristics depending on the people involved. Certain aspects of the content of medical communication share a high degree of consistency across encounters (e.g., history-taking, physical exam[23]). Characteristics like patient age and socioeconomic status have proven to be surprisingly consistent predictors of the ways in which patients and clinicians communicate with each other during the medical encounter.[5] But there are also many differences from one individual encounter to another, such as in the amount and type of humor that is used.[24] Further, the participants' personalities and past experiences, which cannot be changed, are unique factors that the parties bring to the interaction.[5]

In the next section we will address many of the factors that influence the quality and content of the communication (both verbal and nonverbal) that happens in medical settings. As we see in the following analysis, aspects of the physical environment and the events that happen prior to the medical encounter itself can set the stage for the communication between clinician and patient, influencing things like patient participation and later recall. These factors, in turn, influence the individual's commitment to carry out the treatment plans decided during the medical encounter as well as her or his ability to ultimately be successful in doing so.

Physical Environment

Research in the field of business and marketing is rich with studies showing how the physical environment (such as the layout of a shop or the décor in a restaurant) creates an image in the customer's mind about a company or business. Initial impressions are influenced by the atmosphere that a physical environment creates; within that environment, moods, behaviors, and satisfaction with services can be altered.[25-28]

In medical settings, as well, it is increasingly recognized that aspects of the physical environment play an important role. The design and layout of a waiting area and an exam room, including the colors and furnishings, as well as the temperature, noise, and other aspects of the environment can all affect patient satisfaction with care.[29] Characteristics of the medical setting have also been linked to patient anxiety and increased blood pressure.[30] You will recall the effect that high levels of anxiety have on patients' abilities to report, process, and remember information from the medical encounter, so it is important that steps be taken to decrease anxiety if at all possible!

Incorporating a "homelike" design—one that feels familiar—may help patients to be more comfortable,[29, 31, 32] thus reducing their anxiety and increasing their abilities to attend to and remember information. Some evidence that this is true comes from a study in which patients who spent time on a specially designed hospital ward demonstrated better learning about their illness and self-care (as well as higher satisfaction with their care) than did those who spent time on the standard ward.[33] These authors also point out, however, that although patient education on the special ward was more effective, the actual health behaviors following discharge were not significantly different from those of patients who were discharged from the standard ward.

Another environmental feature that has been shown to decrease patient anxiety and physiological reactions (e.g., heightened blood pressure) involves nature scenes. A beautiful and calming view from a window may be very helpful, as might realistic and appropriately lighted pieces of art. Art that depicts water scenes has been found to induce particular calm.[34-36] Aspects of design that are calming and even considered to be healing include on-site gardens, live plants, and structural features that allow natural light to enter a room.[34, 37] Music, too, has been shown to have calming effects on patients.[38]

The degree of privacy that the patient perceives is also important; thus, the way a counseling area is designed can influence the communication between health-care practitioner and patient.[39] Patients should feel that they can speak freely, without being overheard but at the same time the area should not be so small and closed off as to make the patient feel confined. Because most meetings with doctors, nurses, dentists, and physician's assistants take place in private examination or procedure rooms, privacy is usually assured (though sometimes patients do complain about sound traveling through thin walls!). But for other specialties, such as pharmacists, this issue becomes quite salient. More and more frequently, pharmacists are expected to take on some of the educational roles that were previously carried out by other medical professionals. This requires more lengthy discussions, fielding of patient questions, and sometimes even demonstrations of how prescribed medications are to be used. If patients feel that they are exposed or lacking privacy they are likely to hurry through the interaction, paying less attention if they are embarrassed or deciding not to ask some of the questions they may have had.

Some studies show that moods can be influenced by the color of a room's walls; in one study, office workers who spent four days in an office with reddish walls reported feeling more depressed moods than those who spent four days in an office with a blue-green color scheme.[40] It may be that softer colors are similarly more appealing to patients in the health-care setting.

Another study, this one of indoor lighting, found that moods were lowest when participants felt that the lighting was too dark; it got better as light increased up to "just right" and then it decreased again as participants perceived the room as overly bright. An interesting aspect of this study is that when illumination was measured objectively there was no association with mood; all associations were based on personal preferences and perceptions.[27] This research demonstrates just how important individual variation is. In the example at the beginning of this chapter, we saw that Alvin and Sylvia responded differently to Dr. Brenton's interactional style. Individuals in this study of lighting showed that preferences for levels of light were also personal and idiosyncratic.

Another aspect of the physical environment that may affect patients is the health professional's computer in the exam room. This computer may be handheld, laptop, or desktop, and as technology advances, increasing numbers of physicians and medical offices rely on electronic records. More and more offices are moving to computer-based systems. Surveys of patients' perceptions of computers have indicated that patients are generally positive about their use and incorporation into the medical environment.[41] In fact, patients seem to prefer architecture that conveys a sense of "high tech" and instills confidence that the technical aspects of their medical care will be "top-notch."[32] Some research analyzing communication patterns, however, has revealed both positive and negative effects of the presence of computers on the communication process.[42] Being sensitive to whether a patient appreciates such technology or feels threatened or distressed by it, would be important for health-care providers to keep in mind when creating the areas in which they meet with their patients. This caveat is not meant to imply that patients should decide whether computers or electronic medical records are used, because such technology does indeed increase accuracy and reduce medical errors. But the way in which computers are used (for instance, whether a physician has to turn her back to the patient in order to access the records or whether she clearly explains to the patient what she is doing on the computer and why) may be quite important in setting the tone for a medical encounter and thus should not be ignored.

Studies like these suggest that some environmental flexibility might be ideal, so that environments can be tailored to fit the preferences of each patient and to give the patient control and choice.[43] This would not only ensure that patients are as comfortable and relaxed as possible, but also that they are drawn into the role of an active patient.

Here are some examples of ways in which health-care settings can be made more appealing for patients. An interesting toy or two could be added when a child is the patient (being sure to use items that can be disinfected, of course). Lighting could be operated with a dimmer switch, and patients could even be asked to adjust the lights so that they feel most comfortable. Quiet music could be played (or not) as the patient prefers, and the patient could make the musical selection. Chairs could be a type that are easily movable so that different configurations could be achieved, particularly when the patient is accompanied by a family member. Clinicians in various specialty areas will be able to think of other creative ways of making patients feel comfortable, relaxed, and welcomed to join in the health-care partnership.

Verbal Communication

The idea of making medical interviews patient-centered is a popular one, although exactly what is meant by "patient-centered" varies from study to study.[44] Most writers and researchers agree that a patient-centered approach is one that is responsive to the patient's preferences and that views the patient and his or her health from a biopsychosocial perspective rather than from a more narrow, biomedical one.[44–46] It is impossible to know a patient's preferences and psychosocial context, however, without hearing her or his story. Thus, the verbal communication that takes place between patients and their health-care providers is crucial.

Open-ended Questions

One of the most common complaints that patients make is that their medical practitioners don't listen to them[47] and don't ask questions in a format that encourages them to talk. Yet, making a correct diagnosis, finding a treatment plan the patient can adhere to, and connecting with the patient in a meaningful way all require that the health professional listen to the patient, understand the patient's perception of the meaning of his or her symptoms, and know the whole story of the patient's illness experience.[48–50]

Clinical training in medicine emphasizes *differential diagnosis*, in which various possibilities about the causes of symptoms are considered and eliminated, eventually leaving only one, which is then settled on as the "correct" diagnosis. This is much the same as when a biologist "keys out" a questionable animal. The biologist will go, step by step, through a series of simple, dichotomous questions (like "feet webbed or not webbed?") and with each answer, certain possibilities are eliminated. If done correctly, the biologist is led to the correct identification of the specimen. Similarly, a health professional who uses closed-ended questions asks for specific pieces of information using questions that can be answered with "yes" or "no," or with just a word or two. Each question follows another, and each attempts to narrow the range of possibilities until a conclusion is reached.

Although this method, particularly when supplemented with the results of medical tests, can be effective in leading to an appropriate diagnosis, it can also lead the physician to *premature closure*.[51] Premature closure occurs when a diagnosis or other decision is made before all the relevant information is gathered. Using a series of closed-ended questions makes premature closure more likely because the questioner may follow only one path of reasoning, and fail to follow another that might have yielded important information that ultimately changed entirely the diagnosis or decision. An all-too-familiar complaint from clinicians is that their patients suddenly introduce additional symptoms or queries just as the medical visit is nearing completion.[51] The constraints imposed by the exclusive reliance on closed-ended questions from the health professional actually make this more likely to happen. When patients are allowed, on the other hand, to describe their illness experience fully, this problem is much less frequent.[52]

Open-ended questions invite the patient to tell his or her story. These questions are broad, and they rely on the patient to provide pertinent details from which the practitioner can glean what she or he needs to know. For example, a patient's response to "What does the pain feel like to you?" offers the medical professional descriptive material from which he or she can fashion more pointed follow-up questions. When answering open-ended questions, patients are likely to provide a full picture of their experience, and also are likely to describe their symptoms within the psychosocial context in which they have lived those symptoms.[53, 54]

Perhaps, for example, a patient is unsuccessfully struggling to incorporate exercise into his daily schedule. The reason may not be that he can't find the time; he has set aside an hour each day to walk, or go to the gym, or work vigorously in his yard. Instead, his problem may be that he constantly feels fatigued and when it's time to be active, his exhaustion overwhelms him and he simply can't bring himself to do it. What should his clinician make of this? Is the patient simply lazy? Is he suffering from some medical syndrome? Through the telling of his story, the patient might reveal that problems at home preclude him from ever getting a good night's sleep, and in fact his sleep is typically disturbed almost hourly. Addressing this problem then clears the way for the next issue, that of exercising regularly, to be tackled. Thus, for those aiming to provide patient-centered care, the open narrative makes the task easier. In Case Study Box 6.1 we find illustrations of clinician-patient exchanges that differ in terms of the clinician's questioning style and type of information that is shared as a result. These dialogues illustrate the things that may be missed when health professionals rely heavily on closed-ended questions, and the richness of communication that often results when patients are invited to share what they have experienced.

Case Study Box 6.1—Simplified Illustrations of Medical Interviews Using Closed-Ended versus Open-Ended Questions

Medical Problem: Chronic Headaches

Closed-ended Question Dialogue

Physician's Assistant: "So let's discuss these headaches... Would you describe the pain as a stabbing pain?"

Patient: "Yes."

Physician's Assistant: "Is the pain worse in the evening?"

Patient: "Um, sometimes."

Physician's Assistant: "Have you tried over-the-counter pain relievers?"

Patient: "Yeah."

Physician's Assistant: "Which ones have you tried?"

Patient: "Um, I've tried aspirin, and also some 'multisymptom' relief things."

Physician's Assistant: "Have you found that these help?"

Patient: "No, not really."

Physician's Assistant: "Well, maybe you need something stronger. Let's talk about some prescription options, okay?"

Continued

Open-ended Question Dialogue

Physician's Assistant: "So, let's discuss these headaches...Can you describe them to me?"

Patient: "Well, I get them two to four times per week. I'm usually fine in the morning but by midafternoon I can start to feel them coming on. They get pretty severe by late afternoon or evening."

Physician's Assistant: "Describe the pain to me."

Patient: "I'd say that at first it's just a dull ache but as the pain gets worse it starts to throb. It feels like the throbbing almost matches my heartbeat or something. By that point it's not a dull pain anymore, it's much more intense. But it's not sharp."

Physician's Assistant: "And what have you tried to get rid of them, thus far?"

Patient: "Well, I've tried about every pill they have at the drugstore. None of those seem to work very well. Sometimes if I can distract myself when I first start to feel the pain the headache will go away. I usually can't do that though. But two weeks ago I started getting one just as I was packing up to go hiking in the mountains. I would have stayed home but one of my friends was riding with me so I figured I'd give her a ride up, and maybe hike just a little with the group, and make it home before the pain got too bad. But the funny thing was that we were talking in the car, and laughing, and it wasn't until we got up there that I realized the pain was completely gone!"

Physician's Assistant: "Hmmm...it almost sounds like they might be stress-related. You were pretty relaxed when you were driving up to the mountains, right?

Patient: "Yeah."

Physician's Assistant: "Since over-the-counter pain medications don't seem to work for you, I think that you might need something stronger for those times when you can't control the pain. I think you might find a few stress-management techniques useful, too, though. Wouldn't it be great to only have to resort to medications once in a while?"

Refraining from Interruption

Many clinicians seem to have difficulty letting their patients finish what they are saying. One study[51] found that in less than a quarter of the cases studied (23%), patients were allowed to complete their initial statement about what had brought them to the doctor's office. In addition, in more than half the cases, physicians interrupted and directed questions toward one of the specifics the patient had mentioned and this typically happened within the first 18 seconds of the patient's speech. A follow-up study, conducted in 1999, showed a somewhat more positive, but still worrisome, picture in which only 28% of patients were allowed to complete their initial statements of concern, and patients were interrupted after, on average, about 23 seconds instead of 18.[55] Clearly there is still room for improvement.

Failure to listen to a patient's narrative likely sends a message like the following: "I'm in a rush, so please hurry up," or "That second thing you said was important, but the rest of this is not." In addition, interruptions, directions, and failures to listen in medical interviews tell the patient that the health professional is in control and the patient is not. Patients who experience control by their providers tend to have poorer health outcomes and greater levels of dissatisfaction.[21, 56]

As we noted earlier, if providers give their patients too much direction during the medical interview, or interrupt them a great deal, important information can be overlooked. Providers may fail to notice certain important pieces of data from a patient and this can lead to misdiagnoses and medical errors. Or, this information might reemerge near the end of the medical encounter, forcing the clinician to reopen the discussion (possibly throwing off the rest of the clinical schedule) or to delay discussion of the matter until another visit.[51]

An obvious question is, "Will allowing the patient to finish the whole story take up too much time?" Probably not, according to the research findings. Marvel et al.'s study[55] found that patients who were allowed to complete their opening statements took, on average, only about six seconds longer than did those who were interrupted and redirected.

Providing Clear Information

The medical visit clearly involves an *exchange* of information. Health-care providers do more than simply elicit information *from* their patients; they also give information *to* their patients. Communicating effectively with patients requires that verbalizations be thorough and precise, and the patient must be able to understand what is presented to him or her. Thus, it is important that the patient's level of *health literacy* be accurately targeted. This topic was addressed in detail in Chapter 3, as we outlined factors that influence a patient's ability to understand and remember. We noted there how critically important it is for health professionals to clarify with patients what it is that they understand and to define areas where their patients have less knowledge. Then, they should use simple and clear language rather than confusing medical jargon to explain and build on the patient's existing knowledge base. You will recall that when health professionals use technical terms, most of their patients do not comprehend or recall information as well as they do when explanations are less technical in nature.[57] And although studies have shown that the information patients receive varies according to their age, gender, levels of education and anxiety, and the number of questions they ask,[58] it is still vital to   assess   each   individual   patient's   level   of   understanding.   Targeting

communications to the appropriate level is one practical way to promote partnership with patients.[59]

Patients' Verbalizations

Thus far, we have been focusing on the health-care practitioner's verbal communication. The importance of allowing the patient to speak freely has already been
noted, but what factors influence what a patient says? How can the best information
possible be gleaned from a patient's words?

In Chapter 2 we discussed how a patient's beliefs about health, along with
cultural and social factors that influence those beliefs, are important to consider in understanding his or her decisions about health behaviors. These same
variables influence the patient's behavior within the medical interaction. Thus,
eliciting the patient's verbal explanations for symptoms and illness is crucial to
effective communication about health issues and their management—not only
to identify environmental contributors to the problem as in the example above,
but also to help the provider frame health information and interventions in a
way that is most effective for individual patients.[60, 61] For example, a clinician
might ask questions about what the patient thinks has caused the medical
problem, why it might have started at the time it did, or what kind of
treatment might be desired. The patient's answers may provide insight as to
possible causes for the problem, as we saw in the first case study box on open-
ended questions. These answers may also reveal important information that is
relevant to promoting the patient's ultimate adherence. For example, a patient
might say that she does not like to take any medication; the choice of non-
pharmacological remedies (if available) might better address patient preferences and improve patient adherence. If medications must be used,
additional time in discussion with the patient might increase adherence, but
this would not be known if the patient's wariness about medications was not
identified.

Another aspect of the way a patient tells his or her story warrants attention. Somaticizers (also called somatizers), or patients whose symptoms cannot
be directly linked to an organic cause and who convert their emotional distress
to the report of solely physical symptoms, have been found to describe their
symptoms using the same terms and with the same degree of emotion as other
patients. However, they tend not to tell a chronological story of their experience.[62] This is, of course, only one potential clue, but may be an important one
in understanding the patient. Case Study Box 6.2 illustrates the differences with
two hypothetical descriptions from patients, one of them a somaticizer.

Thus, in addition to health-related details that the patient's narrative provides,
the way in which the narrative is told may also provide useful information to the
clinician about the nature of the patient's symptoms and the context surrounding
those symptoms, which might be very useful to know when considering treatment

---

Case Study Box 6.2—Chronological Story Development in Two Patients

Consider the responses of Martin and Renee to the following question, posed by their physical therapist, "How has your back been since your last visit?"

Martin: "I've still been in a lot of pain. My back feels tight and it's like the pain radiates out from about waist-level. It's kind of a tight, squeezing sensation. Sometimes it's not too bad and I can just take my meds and go on with life, but other times I feel like I can't even do my stretches or my exercises. It's just too painful to even start. At that point I just lay down, take a couple of extra pills and hope that it goes away."

Renee: "I've still been in a lot of pain. After our last session I felt better for a couple of days, but then on about the third day I noticed that the pain was significantly worse. It starts out with just some stiffness in the morning but throughout the day a kind of tight, squeezing sensation begins and it gets more and more intense throughout the day. By evening it's radiating out from my lower back, about waist-level, and it's so painful that I can't even do the stretches and exercises I'm supposed to do. Each day it seems like the pinnacle of pain is a little worse. Yesterday and the day before I just had to lay down and take some extra pills."

Both Martin and Renee are describing almost identical symptoms. Yet Renee organizes her description of how her back has been since her last visit with the physical therapist according to the time frame in which her symptoms are experienced, whereas Martin focuses his description of symptoms on the theme, rather than providing a timeline. The chronological development that characterizes Renee's telling (and which is missing from Martin's) suggests that Martin's symptoms, but not likely Renee's, may be interwoven with emotional issues.[62] This provides an important clue that the route to successful symptom management may be different for these two patients.

---

options. For example, one study showed that patients who come to the doctor's office with somatic symptoms of psychological distress will usually talk about the psychological issue *if they are asked*.[63] This is very important because knowing about psychological comorbidities allows the clinician to help (or refer) the patient to alleviate them and/or design medical interventions that take these into account.[64, 65]

Nonverbal cues, of course, can also be quite helpful in identifying patients' unstated emotional distress and other medically relevant issues as well. They are the topic of the next section.

Nonverbal Communication

Much of what is communicated in the medical interaction is actually not said out loud. Instead facial expressions, posture, body movements, voice tone, and other *non*verbal cues are used to convey messages between physician and patient. The sending of these messages is referred to as "encoding," whereas the detection and interpretation of nonverbal signals is called "decoding." For most nonverbal cues, there is no clear and unambiguous meaning. Exceptions include nonverbal symbols, such as the "thumbs up" sign, of course, but even these can vary from culture to culture. Thus, despite the fact that nonverbal cues are used constantly in our social interactions, this subtle yet important language is, just like verbal communication, subject to misunderstanding and errors.

Sometimes nonverbal messages supplement what is said verbally; at other times, verbal and nonverbal messages contradict each other. Take, for example, the case of Julia. When Tina, the office nurse, comes into the examining room to ask a few questions and take vital signs, Julia smiles and cheerfully assures her that everything is just fine and that this should be nothing more than a quick, routine check-up. Tina observes, however, that Julia's movements seem tentative, and when she raises her arm for the blood pressure cuff, Tina catches her wincing a little. She asks, "Did I pinch you?" and Julia shakes her head and intensifies her smile saying, "Oh no, not at all!" Nevertheless, Tina makes a brief notation in the chart so that the physician can follow up during his visit with her. What Julia is not reporting (but her body is) may be important.

Unlike Julia, Miles reports to his physician a rather long list of side effects that he's noticed since beginning a new antidepressant medication. He seems anxious not to leave anything out. Although she is listening intently to his narrative, Dr. Trask also notes several things that Miles hasn't mentioned, including his dilated pupils and a slight tremor in his hands. After asking some follow-up questions and coupling Miles's responses with what she has observed in his nonverbal behavior, Dr. Trask is able to rule out several possible diagnoses and orders some tests in order to narrow the possibilities down even further. In this case, nonverbal cues provide additional, complementary information to what Miles is reporting to his physician. Julia's nonverbal cues provide a cautionary indicator that Julia is not being entirely candid about the symptoms she is experiencing, and this lack of candor may provide a useful hint about Julia's psychosocial context. The conclusions based on their verbal messages would have been different for both of these patients compared with the conclusions reached when also considering their nonverbal communications.

Indicators of Distress

Often patients are reluctant to express emotional discomfort or anxiety about their medical experiences. Some may feel intimidated or think there is not enough time to share their concerns with their health-care professionals. In such situations, patients often express their feelings and emotional experience through nonverbal channels.[15] For example, verbally a patient may say, "I understand," or, "No, I can't think of any questions," but this may not be the complete truth.[66, 67] They may display a confused facial expression or fail to meet the gaze of their health-care provider. The clinician who is alert to these cues may be better prepared to ask the kinds of pointed questions that will elicit needed information and offer reassurances that will result in the patient's decreased anxiety.

Physical Pain and Sensitivity Cues

It has been suggested that level of pain may be best determined nonverbally,[68] and especially for populations that have difficulty with verbal expression (such as preverbal infants and cognitively impaired individuals), observational pain instruments may be necessary.[69] For most people of all ages, nonverbal pain behaviors usually include grimacing, moans, sighs, or clenching. In particular, facial expressions can be useful indicators of physical pain.[70] Although some of our facial expressions can be controlled and manipulated quite well,[71] the cortical pathways that control purposeful facial expressions are different from the subcortical areas that govern spontaneous expressions.[72] Thus, even when consciously trying to "present" certain facial expressions, other facial expressions are likely to "leak" (that is, slip through unintentionally). An astute observer of facial expressions can often obtain a more accurate picture of an individual's experience than one who relies only on the individual's words.

Can one become better at decoding nonverbal messages? To some degree, yes. Although there is variability in the degree to which individuals are naturally attentive to, and accurate in reading, nonverbal cues, there is also evidence that with practice these skills can be increased. Some measurement tools exist that can highlight areas of strength and weakness with regard to nonverbal communication skills. For example, the Profile of Nonverbal Sensitivity (PONS)[73] is a tool that provides subscale scores indicating whether, for example, the individual is good at reading faces or bodies, effective in interpreting variations in tone and inflection in speech, and so on. As another example, Paul Ekman's Facial Action Coding System[74] measures individual abilities to "read" facial expressions but does not address other aspects of nonverbal communication (e.g., body or extralinguistic cues).

Nonverbal skills are sometimes part of communication training programs[75, 76] and training in skills such as empathy with both verbal and nonverbal components has been shown to increase the communication abilities of those who participate in skills training programs.[77]

Desire for Information and Involvement

Many patients want to be involved in their own medical care but don't know how to make their wishes known. If they do recognize what they could do, verbally, to assert their needs, they may be too timid or uncomfortable to do so.[15, 78] Many patients truly desire more information and communication from their physicians but instead of stating this directly, they use indirect tactics such as fidgeting on the examination table to signal their wishes.[79, 80] Smiling, nodding, and leaning forward may all express a desire to be an active participant in the medical care process,[81] and studies show that patients who make little eye contact and hold their bodies in a more closed position (e.g., crossed arms and legs) are less likely to be active participants in their own medical care.[21]

Medically Relevant Information

Because in most medical interactions patients have less power and status than their providers (especially physicians), they are likely to be particularly attentive to the nonverbal cues of their medical care providers. By paying attention to nonverbal cues, patients may garner information without having to ask too many direct questions.[82–84] They may, for example, seek nonverbal information about how well their treatment is progressing.[85] Nonverbal messages have been shown to be especially important in situations where verbal content is suspect (such as when patients think that a dreaded diagnosis is being hidden from them) or difficult to understand (such as when patients don't comprehend some of the medical terms and explanations that members of the health-care team use).[86] Health-care providers must recognize that they are communicating with their patients along two dimensions: the explicitly stated, verbal dimension and the unstated, nonverbal dimension. To achieve this goal, physician training programs in nonverbal communication are being created and refined.[87]

Negotiating the Relationship

Medical staff members often exert control over the medical interaction indirectly, using nonverbal signals. Readiness, on the part of the doctor, to hear the patient's concerns is typically indicated by turning and looking at the patient (body orientation and gaze).[88] Affiliative behaviors such as leaning forward, nodding the head, and smiling indicate to the patient that the practitioner is engaged and interested in what the patient is saying. It suggests to the patient that she or he is encouraged to participate in the medical care process.[84] These behavioral invitations are not inconsequential. Open body posture, smiling and nodding, forward lean, and appropriate gaze have all been linked to improved patient understanding and satisfaction, as well as to decreased anxiety on the part of patients.[20, 89, 90] Table 6.2 provides a sampling of nonverbal behaviors that clinicians may use with their patients to

Table 6.2 Some common nonverbal cues and interpretations relevant to adherence and health behavior change.

Nonverbal domain	Nonverbal cue	Relevance to adherence/behavior change
Facial expression	Smiling	Indicates approval of behavior or liking for patient
	Furrowed brow	Indicates concern, shows empathy
Gaze	Making eye contact with the patient at appropriate times	Shows that the clinician is listening and attentive to their concerns
	Failing to make appropriate eye contact	Signals to patient that clinician is not engaged, or is in a hurry
Posture and body orientation	Facing the patient and leaning forward	Shows that the clinician is focused and desires to collaborate with patient
	Uncrossed arms and legs	Signals relaxation, indicates that clinician is listening, not rushed
Body movement	Fidgeting	Conveys sense of time urgency, impatience
	Touching	Comforts and encourages; invites the patient to a partnership
Voice tone	Warm, supportive and encouraging voice tone	Provides encouragement to overcome the challenges of adhering or changing behavior

convey particular meanings without directly stating them. Although, as noted previously, nonverbal cues can be somewhat ambiguous, we provide likely interpretations and typical ways in which these nonverbal messages are decoded as evidenced by the research literature on this topic.

When both parties in an interaction are attuned to one another, a rhythmic pattern of simultaneous movement takes place, much like a synchronous, nonverbal dance.[91] This synchronous behavior is associated with other positive communication behaviors[92] and seems to be a marker of healthy collaborative relationships, influencing patient outcomes through the shared discussion and decision-making that it fosters. Thus, just as verbal interactivity and the sharing of spoken information are crucial to health promotion,[93, 94] so are coordinated nonverbal exchanges a necessary part of medical relationships that lead to good health behaviors.

Empathy

"Empathy" describes what happens when one identifies with and understands, on a deep level and without judgment, the experience of another. (Note that this is different from sympathy, which denotes that one feels sorry for another.) It is a central concept for psychologists in therapeutic settings, and for medical communicators as well.[95] Saying to someone that you "feel what they are feeling" or that you can "identify with" their experience probably isn't very convincing—empathy is better conveyed through nonverbal means.[90, 91] One task of the medical professional, therefore, is to correctly perceive the patient's inner experience through her or his nonverbal (as well as verbal) cues and to respond in ways that make the patient feel valued and cared for.[96] This happens through many of the channels that indicate attentiveness such as forward lean, open posture, good eye contact, and nodding. Touch is also a common way of reassuring patients and conveying comfort and caring to them.[97]

But empathy can also be conveyed through paralinguistic cues—those that accompany spoken language—such as voice tone and the behavior of "back-channeling." Back-channeling, often identified with an active listening style, refers to those extraverbal utterances that serve to facilitate a narrative but do not interfere with it.[98] For example, as a patient describes the symptoms he's experienced over the past week, the nurse may periodically say things like, "Mmmm-hmmm," "Oh, I see," or "Ah," which indicate to the patient that he is not only being heard but also understood. These utterances are also referred to in the linguistics literature as "continuers." They encourage patients to continue speaking and indicate interest on the part of the listener. By indicating concern and interest, a nurse can convey connection with and *empathy* for the patient.

Although empathic words are often used, voice tone may be just as important in conveying empathy to someone.[99] Warm voice tones are associated with higher degrees of patient satisfaction,[100] but physicians' positive *words* coupled with vocal (but nonverbal) indicators of anxiety or anger are also related positively to patient satisfaction, probably because that combination conveys concern and caring for the patient.[101] Voice tone is related to a number of other health-care outcomes. One of the earliest studies conducted in a medical care setting examined how physicians' voice tone was related to their ability to appropriately refer alcoholic patients for further treatment; specifically, physicians with angry voice tone were less likely to successfully refer these patients.[102] Another study involving ratings of surgeons found that those whose voice tones were judged to be more dominant and less concerned were more likely to have a history of malpractice claims than those who sounded more concerned and collaborative.[103]

Individuals differ somewhat in their natural ability to both understand and express nonverbal information, so the concerned health professional, who wants to serve patients optimally, might ask, "Am I empathic?" or, "Is it possible to learn to be empathic?" The first question is a good one, and the answer probably depends somewhat on the individual's area of specialty. If we had to play the odds, though, our guess would be that many health professionals are not as empathic as they could be. For instance, one particularly poignant study of physician-patient interactions showed that most cues given by patients indicating that they needed empathy (a total of 384 in this study) seemed not to be noticed by physicians (they responded to only 10% of them).[104] As we noted earlier, however, some specialties in health care have counseling and educating as their primary aims—and the focus of much of their training—so it is not surprising to see that empathy rates are somewhat higher in those cases, though still tending to be low.[105] For individuals who are wondering about their own empathy levels, it is indeed possible to measure empathic abilities and also to enhance empathic skills with training and effort.[106, 107] Empathy assessment tools come in different forms, but some of the simplest to use are brief questionnaires. For example, the Jefferson Scale of Physician Empathy is both brief (20 self-report items) and psychometrically sound, predicting empathy in the clinical setting, as rated by supervisors, three years later.[108]

Those desiring to improve their empathy scores might consider a training program.[107, 109] These typically highlight three components: *(1) cognitive* (learning to observe and understand the meaning, at least intellectually, of what is observed in a patient's struggles); *(2) affective*, or emotional (learning to relate observed patient emotions to one's own emotional experience as a way of better connecting with the patient); and *(3) communicative* (learning to effectively convey this cognitive and emotional understanding to the patient).

Conclusion

Forming a relationship with another human being is not always easy, particularly when the interaction is limited in time and largely dictated by the pressing health concerns of one of the parties. Nonetheless, most patients require that strong and collaborative relationships must be formed under just these circumstances if they are to succeed in achieving their health goals. It is important to recognize that many of the factors important in practitioner-patient communication that have been described in this chapter are also applicable to relationships between members of the health-care team, as both types of relationships have great implications for patients' health and well-being. In this chapter we have reviewed typical practitioner-patient relationships, and the roles each individual plays according to the relationship model. We have also evaluated the medical exchange and the factors that influence it, including the physical environment, the ways in which information is sought, and the nonverbal cues that provide a constant backdrop to what is said verbally. Recognizing that time is almost always in short supply (ask any patient or any health professional!), in Chapter 7 we focus on strategies specifically aimed at making medical encounters as efficient as they can possibly be.

References

1. Adewuyi-Dalton R, Ziebland S, Grunfeld E, Hall A. Patients' views of routine hospital follow-up: a qualitative study of women with breast cancer in remission. Psycho-Oncology. 1998;7(5):436–9.
2. Gardner W, Kelleher KJ, Wasserman R, Childs G, Nutting P, Lillienfeld H, Pajer K. Primary care treatment of pediatric psychosocial problems: A study from pediatric research in office settings and ambulatory sentinel practice network. Pediatrics. 2000 Oct;106(4):E44.
3. Krantz DS, Baum A, Wideman M. Assessment of preferences for self-treatment and information in health care. J Pers Soc Psychol 1980;39(5):977–90.
4. Emanuel EJ, Emanuel LL. Four models of the physician-patient relationship. JAMA. 1992;267(16):2221–6.
5. Roter DL, Hall JA. Doctors Talking with Patients/Patients Talking with Doctors: Improving Communication in Medical Visits, 2nd ed. Westport, CT: Greenwood Publishing Group; 2006.
6. Parsons T. The Social System. Glencoe, IL: The Free Press; 1951.
7. Beisecker AE, Beisecker TD. Using metaphors to characterize doctor-patient relationships: paternalism versus consumerism. Health Commun. 1993;5:41–58.
8. Charles C, Gafni A, Whelan T. Decision-making in the physician-patient encounter: revisiting the shared treatment decision-making model. Soc Sci Med. 1999 Sep;49(5):651–61.
9. Coulter A. Paternalism or partnership? Patients have grown up—and there's no going back. BMJ. 1999 Sep 18;319(7212):719–20.
10. Beisecker AE. Aging and the desire for information and input in medical encounters: patient consumerism in medical encounters. The Gerontologist. 1988;28:330–5.
11. Benbassat J, Pilpel D, Tidhar M. Patients' preferences for participation in clinical decision making: a review of published surveys. Behav Med. 1998 Summer;24(2):81–8.
12. Roter DL, Hall JA, Katz NR. Relations between physicians' behaviors and analogue patients' satisfaction, recall, and impressions. Med Care. 1987 May;25(5):437–51.
13. Cornacchia HJ, Barrett S. Consumer Health: A Guide to Intelligent Decisions. St. Louis, MO: Mosby; 1980.
14. Roter DL, Stewart M, Putnam SM, Lipkin M, Jr., Stiles W, Inui TS. Communication patterns of primary care physicians. JAMA. 1997 Jan 22–29;277(4):350–6.
15. Beisecker AE, Beisecker TD. Patient information-seeking behaviors when communicating with doctors. Med Care. 1990 Jan;28(1):19–28.
16. Ballard-Reisch DS. A model of participative decision making for physician-patient interaction. Health Commun. 1990;2(2):91–104.
17. Quill TE, Brody H. Physician recommendations and patient autonomy: finding a balance between physician power and patient choice. Ann Intern Med. 1996 Nov 1;125(9):763–9.
18. Stewart M, Brown JB, Donner A, McWhinney IR, Oates J, Weston WW, Jordan J. The impact of patient-centered care on outcomes. J Fam Pract. 2000 Sep;49(9):796–804.
19. Lussier MT, Richard C. Because one shoe doesn't fit all: a repertoire of doctor-patient relationships. Can Fam Physician. 2008 Aug;54(8):1089–92, 96–9.
20. Beck RS, Daughtridge R, Sloane PD. Physician-patient communication in the primary care office: a systematic review. J Am Board Fam Pract. 2002 Jan–Feb;15(1):25–38.

21. Kaplan SH, Greenfield S, Ware JE, Jr. Assessing the effects of physician-patient interactions on the outcomes of chronic disease. Med Care. 1989 Mar;27(3 Suppl):S110–27.
22. Ong LM, de Haes JC, Hoos AM, Lammes FB. Doctor-patient communication: a review of the literature. Soc Sci Med. 1995 Apr;40(7):903–18.
23. Stiles WB. Stability of the verbal exchange structure of medical consultations. Psychology & Health. 1996;11(6):773–85.
24. Francis L, Monahan K, Berger C. A laughing matter: The use of humor in medical interactions. Motivation and Emotion. 1999; 23(2):155–74.
25. Baker CF. Effect of noise in ICU on heart rate and annoyance in adult postoperative patients. Journal of the American Acoustical Society. 1987; 81(S1): s48.
26. Bitner MJ. Evaluating service encounters: the effects of physical surroundings and employee responses. Journal of Marketing. 1990;54:69–82.
27. Kuller R, Ballal S, Laike T, Mikellides B, Tonello G. The impact of light and colour on psychological mood: a cross-cultural study of indoor work environments. Ergonomics. 2006 Nov 15;49(14):1496–507.
28. Rapoport A. The Meaning of the Built Environment. Beverly Hills, CA: Sage Publications; 1982.
29. Malkin J. Medical and Dental Space Planning. 3rd ed. New York: John Wiley & Sons; 2002.
30. Ulrich RS. Effects of health facility interior design on wellness: theory and recent scientific research. Journal of Health Care Design. 1991; 3:97–109.
31. Martin DP, Hunt JR, Hughes-Stone M, Conrad DA. The Planetree Model Hospital Project: an example of the patient as partner. Hosp Health Serv Adm. 1990 Winter;35(4):591–601.
32. Nesmith EL. Health Care Architecture: Designs for the Future. Washington, DC: American Institute of Architects Press; 1995.
33. Martin DP, Diehr P, Conrad DA, Davis JH, Leickly R, Perrin EB. Randomized trial of a patient-centered hospital unit. Patient Educ Couns. 1998 Jun;34(2):125–33.
34. Miller KM. Planning, Design, and Construction of Health Care Facilities. Joint Commission Resources; 2006.
35. Ulrich RS. Natural versus urban scenes: Some psychophysiological effects. Environment and Behavior. 1981;13:523–56.
36. Ulrich RS. How design impacts wellness. Health Care Forum Journal. 1992 September/October;20–25.
37. Heerwagen JH, Heerwagen DR. Lighting and psychological comfort. Lighting Design + Application. 1986;6:47–51.
38. White JM. Music therapy: an intervention to reduce anxiety in the myocardial infarction patient. Clin Nurse Spec. 1992 Summer;6(2):58–63.
39. Allan EL, Suchanek-Hudmon KL, Berger BA, Eiland SA. Patient treatment adherence. Facility design and counseling skills. J Pharm Technol. 1992 Nov–Dec;8(6):242–51.
40. Kwallek N, Woodson H, Lewis CM, Sales C. Impact of three interior color schemes on worker mood and performance relative to individual environmental sensitivity. Color Research & Application. 1998;22(2):121–32.
41. Houston TK, Ray MN, Crawford MA, Giddens T, Berner ES. Patient perceptions of physician use of handheld computers. AMIA Annu Symp Proc. 2003:299–303.
42. Makoul G, Curry RH, Tang PC. The use of electronic medical records: communication patterns in outpatient encounters. J Am Med Inform Assoc. 2001 Nov–Dec;8(6):610–5.

43. Devlin AS, Arneill AB. Health care environments and patient outcomes: a review of the literature. Environment and Behavior. 2003;35(5):665–94.
44. Mead N, Bower P. Patient-centredness: a conceptual framework and review of the empirical literature. Soc Sci Med. 2000 Oct;51(7):1087–110.
45. Laine C, Davidoff F. Patient-centered medicine. A professional evolution. JAMA. 1996 Jan 10;275(2):152–6.
46. Stewart MB, Brown JB, Weston WW, McWhinney IR, McWilliam CL, Freeman TR. Patient-centered Medicine: Transforming the Clinical Method. Thousand Oaks, CA: Sage Publications; 1995.
47. Probst JC, Greenhouse DL, Selassie AW. Patient and physician satisfaction with an outpatient care visit. J Fam Pract. 1997 Nov;45(5):418–25.
48. Kleinman A. The illness narratives: suffering, healing and the human condition. New York: Basic Books; 1988.
49. Platt FW, Gaspar DL, Coulehan JL, Fox L, Adler AJ, Weston WW, Smith RC, Stewart M. "Tell me about yourself": The patient-centered interview. Ann Intern Med. 2001 Jun 5;134(11):1079–85.
50. Smith RC, Hoppe RB. The patient's story: integrating the patient- and physician-centered approaches to interviewing. Ann Intern Med. 1991 Sep 15;115(6):470–7.
51. Beckman HB, Frankel RM. The effect of physician behavior on the collection of data. Ann Intern Med. 1984 Nov;101(5):692–6.
52. Barrier PA, Li JT, Jensen NM. Two words to improve physician-patient communication: what else? Mayo Clin Proc. 2003 Feb;78(2):211–4.
53. Haidet P, Paterniti DA. "Building" a history rather than "taking" one: a perspective on information sharing during the medical interview. Arch Intern Med. 2003 May 26;163(10):1134–40.
54. Levinson W, Gorawara-Bhat R, Lamb J. A study of patient clues and physician responses in primary care and surgical settings. JAMA. 2000 Aug 23–30;284(8):1021–7.
55. Marvel MK, Epstein RM, Flowers K, Beckman HB. Soliciting the patient's agenda: have we improved? JAMA. 1999 Jan 20;281(3):283–7.
56. Hall JA, Irish JT, Roter DL, Ehrlich CM, Miller LH. Satisfaction, gender, and communication in medical visits. Med Care. 1994 Dec;32(12):1216–31.
57. Jackson LD. Information complexity and medical communication: the effects of technical language and amount of information in a medical message. Health Commun. 1992;4(3):197–210.
58. Street R. Information-giving in medical consultations: The influence of patients' communicative styles and personal characteristics. Soc Sci Med. 1991;32(5):541–8.
59. Schillinger D, Piette J, Grumbach K, Wang F, Wilson C, Daher C, Leong-Grotz K, Castro C, Bindman AB. Closing the loop: physician communication with diabetic patients who have low health literacy. Arch Intern Med. 2003 Jan 13;163(1):83–90.
60. Betancourt JR, Carrillo JE, Green AR. Hypertension in multicultural and minority populations: linking communication to compliance. Curr Hypertens Rep. 1999 Dec;1(6):482–8.
61. Kleinman A, Eisenberg L, Good B. Culture, illness, and care: clinical lessons from anthropologic and cross-cultural research. Ann Intern Med. 1978 Feb;88(2):251–8.
62. Elderkin-Thompson V, Silver RC, Waitzkin H. Narratives of somatizing and nonsomatizing patients in a primary care setting. J Health Psychol. 1998;3(3):407–28.

63. Robinson JW, Roter DL. Psychosocial problem disclosure by primary care patients. Soc Sci Med. 1999 May;48(10):1353–62.
64. Anfinson TJ, Bona JR. A health services perspective on delivery of psychiatric services in primary care including internal medicine. Med Clin North Am. 2001 May;85(3):597–616.
65. Bertakis KD, Callahan EJ, Azari R, Robbins JA. Predictors of patient referrals by primary care residents to specialty care clinics. Fam Med. 2001 Mar;33(3):203–9.
66. Cormier L, Cormier WH, Weisser, RJ. Interviewing and Helping Skills for Health Professionals. Belmont, CA: Wadsworth; 1984.
67. Patterson ML. Nonverbal Behavior: A Functional Perspective. New York: Springer-Verlag; 1983.
68. Craig KD, Prkachin KM, Grunau RVE. The facial expression of pain. In: Turk DC, Melzack R, editors. Handbook of Pain Assessment. New York: Guilford; 2001.
69. Feldt KS. The checklist of nonverbal pain indicators (CNPI). Pain Manag Nurs. 2000 Mar;1(1):13–21.
70. Prkachin KM, Craig KD. The communication and interpretation of facial pain signals. J Nonverbal Behav. 1995;19(4):191–205.
71. Ekman P, Friesen WV. Detecting deception from the body or face. J Pers Soc Psychol. 1974;29(3):288–98.
72. Rinn WE. Neuropsychology of facial expression. In: Feldman RS, Rimer B, editors. Fundamentals of nonverbal behavior. Cambridge, UK: Cambridge University Press; 1991.
73. Rosenthal R, Hall JA, DiMatteo MR, Rogers PL, Archer D. Sensitivity to Nonverbal Communication: The PONS Test. Baltimore, MD: Johns Hopkins University Press; 1979.
74. Ekman P, Friesen WV, Hager JC. The Facial Action Coding System, 2nd ed. London: Weidenfeld & Nicolson; 2002.
75. Kurtz SM, Silverman J, Draper J. Teaching and Learning Communication Skills in Medicine. Abingdon, Oxon, UK: Radcliffe Medical Press; 2005.
76. Mast MS. On the importance of nonverbal communication in the physician-patient interaction. Patient Educ Couns. 2007 Aug;67(3):315–8.
77. Roter DL, Hall JA, Kern DE, Barker LR, Cole KA, Roca RP. Improving physicians' interviewing skills and reducing patients' emotional distress. A randomized clinical trial. Arch Intern Med. 1995 Sep 25;155(17):1877–84.
78. Haug M,Lavin B. Consumerism in Medicine. Beverly Hills, CA: Sage; 1983.
79. Blanchard CG, Labrecque MS, Ruckdeschel JC, Blanchard EB. Information and decision-making preferences of hospitalized adult cancer patients. Soc Sci Med. 1988;27(11):1139–45.
80. Heath C. Talk and recipiency: Sequential organization in speech and body movement. In: Atkinson JM, Heritage J, editors. Structures of Social Action: Studies in Conversation Analysis. Cambridge, UK: Cambridge University Press; 1984.
81. Coker DA, Burgoon J. The nature of conversational involvement and nonverbal encoding patterns. Hum Commun Res. 1987;13(4):463–94.
82. DiMatteo MR, DiNicola DD. Achieving Patient Compliance: The Psychology of the Medical Practitioner's Role. New York: Pergamon Press; 1982.
83. Fiske ST. Controlling other people. The impact of power on stereotyping. Am Psychol. 1993; 48(6):621–8.
84. Lepper HS, Martin LR, DiMatteo MR. A model of nonverbal exchange in physician-patient expectations for patient involvement. J Nonverb Behav. 1995; 19(4):207–22.

85. Friedman HS. Nonverbal communication in medical interaction. In: Friedman HS, DiMatteo MR, editors. Interpersonal Issues in Health Care. New York: Academic Press; 1982.
86. DePaulo BM, Friedman HS. Nonverbal communication. In: Gilbert D, Fiske S, Lindzey G, editors. Handbook of Social Psychology. 4th ed. Boston: McGraw Hill; 1998. p. 3–40.
87. Martin L, Friedman HS. Nonverbal communication and health care. In: Riggio RE, Feldman RS, editors. Applications of Nonverbal Communication. Mahwah, NJ: Lawrence Erlbaum; 2005. p. 3–16.
88. Robinson JD. Getting down to business: talk, gaze, and body orientation during openings of doctor-patient consultations. Hum Commun Res. 1998;25(1):97–123.
89. Ambady N, Koo J, Rosenthal R, Winograd CH. Physical therapists' nonverbal communication predicts geriatric patients' health outcomes. Psychol Aging. 2002 Sep;17(3):443–52.
90. Harrigan JA, Oxman TE, Rosenthal R. Rapport expressed through nonverbal behavior. J Nonverb Behav. 1985 9(2):95–110.
91. Hall JA, Harrigan JA, Rosenthal R. Nonverbal behavior in clincian patient interaction. Appl Prev Psychol. 1995;4(1):21–37.
92. Koss T, Rosenthal R. Interactional synchrony, positivity, and patient satisfaction in the physician-patient relationship. Med Care. 1997 Nov;35(11):1158–63.
93. Neuhauser L, Kreps G. Rethinking communication in the e-health Era. J Health Psychol. 2003;8(1):7–23.
94. Street RJ, Rimal R. Health promotion and interactive technology: A conceptual foundation. In: RL Street Jr, Gold W, Manning T, editors. Health promotion and interactive technology: Theoretical applications and future directions. Mahwah, NJ: Lawrence Erlbaum; 1997. p. 1–18.
95. Cormier SL, Cormier WH, Weisser RJ. Interviewing and Helping Skills for Health Professionals. Monterey, CA: Wadsworth Health Sciences Division; 1984.
96. Colliver J, Willis, MS, Robbs, RS, Cohen, DS, Swartz, MH. Applied research: assessment of empathy in a standardized-patient examination. Teach Learn Med. 1998;10:8–11.
97. Blondis MN, Jackson BE. Nonverbal Communication with Patients. New York: Wiley & Sons; 1977.
98. Duncan S. On the structure of speaker-auditor interaction during speaker turns. Language in Society. 1974;2:161–80.
99. Tickle-Degnen LG, Gavett E. Changes in nonverbal behavior during the development of therapeutic relationships. In: P. Philippot, Feldman RS, Coats EJ, editors. Nonverbal Behavior in Clinical Settings. New York: Oxford; 2003. p. 75–110.
100. Haskard KB, Williams SL, DiMatteo MR, Heritage J, Rosenthal R. The provider's voice: patient satisfaction and the content-filtered speech of nurses and physicians in primary medical care. J Nonverb Behav. 2008;32:1–20.
101. Hall JA, Roter DL, Rand CS. Communication of affect between patient and physician. J Health Soc Behav. 1981 Mar;22(1):18–30.
102. Milmoe S, Rosenthal R, Blane HT, Chafetz ME, Wolf I. The doctor's voice: postdictor of successful referral of alcoholic patients. J Abnorm Psychol. 1967 Feb;72(1):78–84.
103. Ambady N, Laplante D, Nguyen T, Rosenthal R, Chaumeton N, Levinson W. Surgeons' tone of voice: a clue to malpractice history. Surgery. 2002 Jul;132(1):5–9.
104. Morse DS, Edwardsen EA, Gordon HS. Missed opportunities for interval empathy in lung cancer communication. Arch Intern Med. 2008 Sep 22;168(17):1853–8.

105. Reynolds WJ, Scott B. Do nurses and other professional helpers normally display much empathy? J Adv Nurs. 2000 Jan;31(1):226–34.
106. Bertman S, Krant MJ. To know of suffering and the teaching of empathy. Soc Sci Med. 1977 Sep;11(11–13):639–44.
107. Feighny KM, Monaco M, Arnold L. Empathy training to improve physician-patient communication skills. Acad Med. 1995 May;70(5):435–6.
108. Hojat M, Mangione S, Nasca TJ, Gonnella JS, Magee M. Empathy scores in medical schools and ratings of empathic behavior in residency training 3 years later. J of Social Psychology. 2005;145(6):663–72.
109. Fine VK, Therrien ME. Empathy in the doctor-patient relationship: skill training for medical students. J Med Educ. 1977 Sep;52(9):752–7.

7

Effective Collaboration with Patients—On a Tight Schedule

We always have enough time if we will but use it aright.
—Goethe

It is probably not news to you that patients don't usually receive as much time with their physicians as they would like. You may feel that way about your own doctor visits! Less recognized, though, is that many physicians share this concern. For example, the *Community Tracking Study Physician Survey* found that nearly one-third of the 6,628 primary care physicians surveyed during 2004–2005 felt that they did not have adequate time with their patients during most office visits.[1] In addition, about half of all patients leave their doctors' offices without a clear understanding of the information and advice they received.[2, 3]

Brief office visits pose a clear challenge to the delivery of effective health care.[4] With only limited time, and so much to do and discuss, what is the best way to proceed? Keeping in mind the mental checklist of information-motivation-strategy discussed in earlier chapters, we describe here how a division of labor among the members of the health-care team and the utilization of technology can help make the most of medical interactions. In this chapter, we focus on many ways to share information, energize for change, and creatively adjust behavior in order to achieve health goals despite limitations on time.

Importance of the Health-Care Team

Most of the existing research on medical interactions has focused on what happens between patients and their physicians. Of course, in reality medical care involves a number of different providers, and patients may typically spend substantially more time interacting with other members of the medical staff than with their physicians.

The complexity of today's medical care makes functioning without a team-oriented approach nearly impossible for physicians. In addition, efforts to contain health-care costs, while maintaining high quality, encourage organizations to meet certain patient needs with additional clinical staff and caregivers who specialize in areas that fall outside the purview of many physicians.[5-12]

What is a health-care team? A health-care team can be described as a group of clinicians, often diverse, who oversee medical care for a particular patient or group of patients—communicating about and participating in the patient's treatment and the management of his or her conditions.[13] Depending on the nature of the patient's needs, the term *health-care team* might thus mean a variety of different things. For a recently diagnosed but advanced-stage diabetic, the team will likely include at least one physician (perhaps more, if specialists are needed for consultation or treatments), a physician's assistant, nurse, or nurse practitioner, a nutritionist, a medical educator, and a support-staff member to coordinate the patient's care schedule (setting appointments, calling with appointment reminders, and processing paperwork related to the patient's care and reimbursement for that care). For someone whose primary problem is hypertension, the team might include only the primary care physician, and his or her assistant (nurse or medical assistant). The team might ideally also include a specialist in biofeedback or a counselor or social worker to help the individual reduce and manage stress.

Simply having the necessary group members in place, however, does not ensure that they will function in a cohesive, teamlike manner. Thus, a more complete description of the ideal health-care team also involves characteristics of group functioning, including: *(1)* clear and measurable team goals, *(2)* clearly defined systems for accomplishing those goals, *(3)* clear and precise division of tasks, *(4)* adequate training of all team members for their particular tasks, and *(5)* effective communication among the team members (and you will recall that in Chapter 6 we noted that many of the same principles that are important for effective clinician-patient interactions also apply to interactions between health-care team members).[8, 12]

Is the establishment of a well-integrated health-care team one pathway to more effective and efficient medical encounters? Research studies suggest that the answer is "yes." In managing chronic diseases, shared responsibility among primary care physicians and other team members for both medical management and support services has been shown to be quite successful.[12, 14, 15] Patients who are cared for by a cohesive health-care team experience better health outcomes and report higher levels of satisfaction than do those with more fragmented care or who are cared for by a team that fails to communicate effectively.[16-20]

Subpar communication on the part of health-care teams is more than just inefficient, of course. Poor communication can have dire consequences such as increasing the likelihood of medical errors. In particular, verbal communications are susceptible to misunderstanding and misinterpretation, perhaps because they are not already written down and instead must be recalled. Written instructions, on the other hand, can be rechecked when memories need refreshing. Another factor making verbal instructions particularly vulnerable to error is that they are more likely to be given in situations in which people are distracted and hurried (such as in emergencies, or when people are ill or not at their best).[21] The anxiety of the person receiving the verbal communication, as well as the various distractions that may be present in a chaotic situation probably also contribute to making verbal communications especially prone to errors. Setting up protocols for communicating—such as designating ahead of time who is responsible for pursuing, receiving, and, disseminating various types of information and agreeing on a common vocabulary—are methods by which members of the health-care team can make their own communications with one another more accurate and precise.

The concept of agreeing on a common vocabulary may seem unnecessary; after all, don't health professionals all use the same vocabulary anyway? Although this might seem reasonable to assume, it is not the case. Medical textbooks, scientific articles, and technical reports are usually quite precise in their terminology and they are careful to explain how words are being used whenever there is room for ambiguity. They rely almost exclusively on denotations (direct, specific meanings) and strive to avoid connotative usage (meanings that are implied, aside from what is explicitly stated). But in everyday language we often use connotative language, and the medical context is no exception. For example, a nurse who is new to a clinic might report to the physician that Mr. Albertson, who is waiting in the examination room, has eczema. In her previous workplace, many skin conditions were referred to with this general and somewhat ambiguous term. In this clinic, however, eczema is only used to refer to *recurrent skin* rashes that include swelling along with at least one other symptom (e.g., itching, crusting/flaking, blistering, cracking, oozing, or bleeding). Since Mr. Albertson's condition is not recurrent, and his skin is red and slightly swollen but does not itch or exhibit any of the other criteria used by this medical clinic to diagnose eczema, this nurse's colleagues do not consider him to have eczema, but instead to have merely a "rash."

Perhaps even more alarming than the potential for misunderstandings created by variations in connotative meanings is the finding that medical professionals do not always use medical terms appropriately. One study, for example, found that physicians used vocabulary in ways that were technically incorrect about 30 percent of the time.[22] Thus, the recommendation that all team members understand and use a common vocabulary is not a superfluous one. Instead, a common vocabulary assures that communications among team members are as efficient and effective as they can possibly be, thus streamlining the care process.

Although team-delivered care has many benefits, it is not yet widely used. One reason may be that without a full understanding of how people can work together in groups, teams can easily become too large and complex to accomplish their aims efficiently. The sheer effort and coordination required for a team of 15 to work together to care for all the patients in a practice, for example, may outweigh the benefits of the individual specialized and complementary services. It has been suggested that team size may have a U-shaped relationship to effectiveness, with teams that are too small or too large being at a disadvantage.[23] Although it is difficult to say exactly how many members a team should have, it has been suggested that a team comprised of about 6 members is ideal and that teams with 12 or more members are generally too big to work efficiently.[24]

The optimal composition of a health-care team will, of course, be determined by factors that are unique to the situation, including the number and type(s) of patients that are being served. In general, it seems that to maximize cost effectiveness, a team's tasks should be completed by those with the lowest level of training that would equip them for the task. This frees those with higher levels of expertise to focus on tasks that they are specially trained to address.[5] Having tasks completed by those with relatively lower levels of training does not mean that the quality of care suffers. Evidence is good that, for many tasks, the care delivered by a nurse practitioner is equivalent to that delivered by the primary care physician.[25, 26] And, because of their training, nurse practitioners may actually be better at delivering certain kinds of care, especially related to chronic disease management and behavioral counseling.[9, 12]

Another barrier to successful implementation of a team approach is the set of interpersonal challenges that often typify a team environment, including personal conflicts and issues related to power-sharing.[27] Forming teams of people who communicate and work well with each other is crucial to the success of the treatment a health-care team delivers. Just as the communication and partnership between patients and their health-care providers is vital, so is the information-sharing, negotiation, trust, and collaboration among those caring for the patient.

Despite the challenges of implementing coordinated and efficient systems for team-based care, the benefits of having multiple health-care providers functioning as a team appear to outweigh the drawbacks. For a time-strapped physician, there may be great value in being able to rely on a trusted pharmacist to discuss medication details with the patient and an experienced nurse to work with the patient to overcome individual or system-related barriers to adherence. There are many specific strategies for using a team approach or various types of technological advances to help make the most of the usually limited medical visit time. Let us examine these next.

Using Teams and Technology to Deliver Care

Planning the Medical Visit

When Tamara prepares for her upcoming annual exam with her primary care physician, she makes a list of all of her concerns. She has been experiencing low back pain and headaches, she is worried that her blood pressure may be too high, and she wonders whether she should be on medication for hypertension. She has also been struggling with nagging feelings of anxiety (not all related to worrying about her health) that seem to have worsened. Tamara is like many patients who present multiple symptoms and concerns during a single medical visit. The agenda that a patient like Tamara brings to the medical encounter may be quite different from the agenda of the medical staff. Thus, spending time training the medical team to efficiently organize the medical visit in a way that meets both patients' and professionals' needs, can result in tangible benefits to the patient. For instance, one study showed that a brief 90-minute workshop for physicians on how to elicit the patient's agenda and negotiate priorities for the visit resulted in a significant increase in patients' perceptions that all of their concerns had been addressed during the interaction.[28]

In Chapter 3 we discussed memory-enhancement tools, one of which was aimed at helping patients to remember important steps in making medical decisions. This tool, PREPARED®[29], uses an acronym in which each letter indicates a stage in the process of making informed, collaborative choices. Even if a particular task is not directly decision-oriented, however, using a consistent set of procedures to organize a visit and interact with patients may help to assure that important elements of the patient's needs and experience are not overlooked. A reliable routine may also help the patient to feel more comfortable, thus freeing her or his mind to focus on questions that need to be asked or on understanding and remembering what is explained by the health professional.

Preappointment Counseling

If you were to phone a radio talk show, you wouldn't immediately be put on the air. You would first talk with a screener whose job it is to help callers formulate their questions and comments. This way, valuable "air time" wouldn't be wasted with rambling and disjointed communications. Each minute spent in the medical interaction is also vitally important, so planning ahead to use that time efficiently is an effective strategy to employ.

Regardless of the composition of the medical care "team" (physician, medical assistant, and receptionist in a small office; or a group of physicians and other clinicians from various specialties in a larger practice), previsit counseling by either a physician or a nonphysician health-care provider can help set the agenda for the visit.[30] Agenda setting involves organizing which issues have priority so that the most important things are sure to be covered during the visit. This may involve some negotiation, of course, because the patient's priorities may not be the same as those of the clinician). It also involves helping the patient to set reasonable expectations for what will be covered during the encounter and what might need to be deferred until a later visit. And finally, if the agenda is being constructed by someone other than the primary clinician, the patient may need help to organize and formulate any questions that will be asked during the medical visit. This time can also be used to conduct some of the more mundane elements of typical visits, such as verifying the patient's current medications, taking the history, and checking vital signs.[4] Agenda-setting is a critical but often overlooked component of efficient care delivery. Training health-care providers in setting an agenda for the visit can improve the informational skills of the clinician and the quality of the communication process.[31]

Interactive Health Communication (IHC)

Increasingly, people want (or even expect) the achievement of their health-care needs to be convenient. Automated systems for making appointments and checking test results along with downloadable forms that patients can access and complete prior to their appointments may increase efficiency dramatically.[32] Automated, interactive systems are not only convenient, they may also reduce the amount of time it takes to ask appropriate follow-up questions based logically on the responses of the patient[33, 34] and they can serve as very effective educational tools.[35] Automated systems also reduce errors, such as when online prescription systems decrease mistakes in dosage amounts or drug names.[36] Not only can they make prescriptions more accurate, but automated or semiautomated systems can also make adherence easier for patients. For example, most pharmacies now allow refills to be ordered online with details of the previous prescription already filled in on the patient's order form. Other online services can also be useful to patients, such as the provision of information about prescriptions or electronic refill reminders. Table 7.1 summarizes some of the benefits of these services to patients.

With regard to gathering information from patients, some data suggest that patients may be more open to disclosing, and less influenced by social desirability pressures, when responding to a computerized assessment than when interacting in person or over the phone with an interviewer,[34, 37] particularly if the information is embarrassing or the patient believes it portrays him or her in a poor light. For

Table 7.1 Benefits of Online, Automated Pharmacy Systems for Patients

Pharmacy Service	Benefit to Patients
Online Refill Ordering	Increases efficiency for patients, reducing time spent on telephone hold or transportation when ordering in person
Electronic Refill Reminders	Reduces patient forgetfulness; Ensures that patients don't "run out" due to poor planning
Automatic Refills	Reduces patient forgetfulness beyond reductions seen with refill reminders; Decreases delays due to patient "busy-ness"
Medication Information Online	Allows patients to better understand their medications or to easily re-obtain medication information if the hard copy is lost
Delivery by Mail	Reduces the burden associated with obtaining medications, especially for those with transportation difficulties

example, a patient may feel uncomfortable describing problems with sexual functioning or gynecological issues to a clinician of the other gender. Or, perhaps it is easier to check off a list of what one ate yesterday than it is to sit in front of someone else and recount dietary blunders. In these cases the more abstract format of the computerized assessment might decrease emotions such as anxiety or embarrassment, thereby making accurate recall and honest reporting more likely.

Technology may also be used to help reconcile the patient's vocabulary with that of the practitioner, particularly when patients are "answering" questions using an automated system. Lay vocabulary can sometimes be quite different from that of professionals even when the same medical issue is being described.[22, 38] To help address this problem *WellMed Inc.*'s "Consumer Health Terminology" program, for example, maps 20,000 common terms that patients might use to report medical information onto technical terms in SNOMED (Systematized Nomenclature of Medicine) and other databases.[39] Although this particular system is part of a suite of services for *WellMed Inc.*'s consumers (and not publicly available), it nonetheless represents another way in which technology is being developed and used to increase efficiency while optimizing patient health outcomes; systems such as this one are likely to become more prevalent with time.[40, 41]

It is important to keep in mind, however, that automated systems, such as those described above, change the interaction with, but do not reduce the importance of, the health-care team. A patient who accesses laboratory results online may still need to discuss them with a clinician. Educating a patient about behavior change addresses the informational (and perhaps strategy) components of our information-motivation-strategy model but may do little to motivate and does not ensure actual change. And, some types of test results (e.g., those regarding a serious illness or involving complicated data) should *not* be made available electronically but instead should be presented in person and discussed with a physician or other team member.[35] In these cases, where the information is likely to be troubling to the patient, it is desirable to structure the clinical routine so that test results can be received as quickly as possible and to ensure that there is adequate time for their full discussion at that same meeting. For instance, testing for HIV is often done using a rapid format such that patients are able to learn their results and be counseled about them during the same visit.[42]

There are also potential drawbacks associated with using automated systems. In some cases, patients might receive information that is not useful to them, and they may even become frustrated or confused if they interact with the automated system in unanticipated (unprogrammed) ways, such as by seeking information about a health concern that the system is not equipped to handle.[35] Patients may also generalize and believe that all (or much) information that they obtain electronically is reliable or useful whereas in fact, many websites provide erroneous health information.[43] Thus, some guidance will likely be needed before most patients will be able to appropriately use automated systems to meet some of their health-care needs.

Even when communication is done electronically, its form and structure remain important. As noted above, information is not all that is needed for individuals to make health-relevant changes in their lives, and simply providing patients with access to medical information online is not nearly as effective as providing them with more interactive and individualized online resources.[44] For example, one study[45] looked at the effectiveness of providing online education versus online behavioral therapy for weight loss. All participants in this study attended an introductory meeting where they received an hour of training on weight control and learned about using the internet-based materials. Participants were instructed on the importance of self-monitoring and everyone used web-based resources to keep track of their daily diet and exercise throughout the course of the study. Everyone also had two brief follow-up visits with the psychologist, but only the experimental group completed weekly electronic self-monitoring diaries and received feedback on these (in the form of behavioral lessons and individualized encouragement, responses to questions, and strategies/recommendations based on their diaries). Patients in the behavioral therapy group also had access to an online bulletin board on which they could interact with other members of their group. At the end of the 9-month study, analyses showed that those in the behavioral therapy group (which was more individualized) had lost significantly more weight and had maintained their losses (rather than having their weight creep back up over the course of the study, as was seen for the web-based education-only group).

The importance of individualization, or personalizing, has been well demonstrated (in Chapters 3 and 4, as well as in this chapter). Some of the most useful features of electronic communications involve their ability to combine individually tailored content with mass-media style dissemination that can be constantly updated.[46, 47] These interactive media forms are powerful because of their flexibility, and for some patients they have the additional appeal of novelty; that is, some patients find the novelty of these media to be attractive and compelling in their own right, regardless of any other benefits.[48]

For others, however, this constantly changing technology may instead be an obstacle that must be repeatedly overcome (especially for those who have not grown up with electronic communication media such as text messaging, FaceBook, and Twitter), and the inevitable "updates" may render purchased systems quickly obsolete—either because patients become frustrated with them or because the systems become costly to maintain.[35] Despite these potential problems, however, several literature reviews indicate that e-health communications positively influence a wide range of behavioral outcomes, from smoking cessation to management of diabetes and osteoarthritis to increasing physical activity and improving diet.[49-52]

Health communications that involve *interactive* technology are particularly effective. To illustrate, one review of 141 interventions using tailored messages found that telephone-delivered messages were more effective than tailored print material[47] while another study found that combining tailored telephone and tailored print messages was highly effective.[53] A creative example of an even more interactive tool being integrated with the medical visit to improve the efficiency of medical communication is PACE+.[54] This system allows a patient to complete a computer-based application, have activity and nutrition behaviors assessed, and receive suggestions for possible change all while waiting in the reception area. The clinician receives the information before the visit and intervention strategies based on those data are pursued.

Another creative example of IHC is the *Health Buddy* system, which is used for evaluating pediatric asthma symptoms.[55] The *Buddy* device is attached to a home phone and children are asked a series of questions about their symptoms, their use of medications, and the effects of asthma on their functioning. To make it more fun for kids, trivia questions are also included and children's answers receive responses from the device. Their asthma-relevant responses are sent on to a nurse for evaluation and follow-up. Both the *Health Buddy* and *Pace+* systems illustrate the streamlining of medical communication and health-care delivery that can happen with the aid of technology. Let us now turn to some nontechnological methods for improving efficiency in medicine.

Group Consultations

Dr. Bailey specializes in diabetes care. On this Tuesday, she spends about 10 minutes with each of her patients, going over test results and discussing blood glucose management techniques. She must structure her time in each visit carefully so as not to be late for the next appointment. Feelings of guilt arise when one of her patients has questions that she can't take the time to answer. Instead, she asks her patient to schedule another appointment to go over these remaining issues. Dr. Zimmer also provides diabetes care, and on this Tuesday he meets with five of his patients at the same time in a group meeting. (These patients have all agreed to have others know they are working on management of their diabetes and know that although they may choose to share their personal information in the group, Dr. Zimmer will not disclose anything about them to others.) Before the group meeting, he has reviewed all of their test results, and is prepared to follow up with two of the patients after the group meeting for brief one-on-one counseling. The group meeting lasts about 30 minutes and group members share tips and techniques for managing their blood sugar levels, discuss everyday barriers they face in successfully managing their treatment regimens, and provide support for one another. Dr. Zimmer guides the discussion, shares some advice, and provides encouragement. At the end of the session everyone feels that they have benefited from the meeting.

When multiple patients with similar chronic diseases or other shared health issues can be seen together as a group, several positive outcomes are likely. First, because general information only has to be stated once, rather than repeated for each patient, more time is available for discussing issues in depth, or from a variety of perspectives. Also, the multiple viewpoints and experiences that members bring to the group allow creative ideas and strategies for coping with health-related problems to emerge. Finally, the opportunity to interact with others who share similar struggles can be an effective coping aid, giving a sense that there are others "in the same boat" and helping to build the individual patient's confidence through the processes of social comparison and vicarious experience,[56] as we saw with Ardis in Chapter 2.

Patient groups may be led by a physician, or by another member of the health-care team, but in all cases careful thought must be given to the form and function of the group. How many people will comprise the group? Will everyone have the same health issue, and will they be at about the same age and stage in the health-care process? How will group members be recruited? Will the format be mostly lecture-style, a guided discussion, or some combination of the two? Will the same person lead the group at each meeting, or will different individuals take responsibility depending on the topic?

Outcomes associated with such group visits are generally positive. In a randomized trial with older patients, participants in the group consultation were more satisfied with the care they received, more health literate, and they utilized fewer services than did those receiving traditional consultations.[57] In another randomized trial, this time with diabetes patients, those who participated in group visits had lower glycosylated hemoglobin levels, better quality of life, greater understanding about their illness, and better health behaviors than did those who had traditional medical visits.[58]

Technology-Based Decision-Making Aids

Hearing the experiences of others is one benefit of group visits, and getting feedback in a group setting can often be helpful to patients making decisions about their health care. In Chapter 5 we discussed a variety of decision-making aids that can be used to help patients understand the various risks and options associated with their medical condition and possible treatments. Some of these require only simple materials (e.g., paper and pen, or a decision board) but others rely on more sophisticated technology to engage the patient.

Videotapes and DVDs can be used to provide patients with information and a variety of perspectives when there is not enough time in the medical encounter to thoroughly discuss all of them.[59, 60] For example, a brief (22-minute) videotape on prostate-specific antigen (PSA) screening provides balanced information on the test and discusses why one would or would not want to have it. The videotape includes a testimonial from a physician who regularly undergoes PSA screening and another from a physician who chooses not to.[61]

Patients who viewed the videotape were better informed about PSA screening, more satisfied with the information they received, and more interested in collaborating in making medical decisions than were those who did not see the videotape.[62] As an interesting aside, patients who viewed the video were less likely to have the screening; only about 60 percent of the video viewers chose to have screening, compared with 98 percent of those who hadn't seen the video.

Some decision aids are more interactive than a video or DVD presentation, and often these are internet-based. Interactive decision aids allow patients to select additional information on particular subtopics and to control the ordering of information acquisition. They can view educational videos, hear from people who are faced with the same choices, and join support or discussion groups. These options mirror some of those associated with in-person group visits.[63] Depending on the nature of the medical choices they are contemplating, patients may also be able to get tailored information about the likelihoods of various outcomes (such as discussed in Chapter 5). Although individual websites will likely provide only some of these features, studies indicate that patients who use these tools become more actively involved in making medical decisions, feel less conflict about their decisions, and are more satisfied with the information they receive using these tools than when they receive information for making decisions just by consulting with their physicians.[64, 65] Internet-based consumer health-decision support tools, may be superior to simple VHS and DVD audiovisual presentations because their flexibility means that patients who are already well versed in particular aspects of their illness or a treatment do not have to view simpler portions of the information available and can move on to the information at the level where they feel most comfortable. The features of five online decision-making tools (all available to the public) are summarized and compared in Table 7.2.

Follow-Up Management

Patient outcomes, both objective clinical outcomes and self-reported personal experiences, can be improved with consistent follow-up consultation, either from the physician or from another health professional. Research shows that both blood glucose levels and self-reported health were better when patients worked with a nurse case manager, dietitian, and exercise counselor after their initial consultations than when they received just standard care (mostly encouragement to self-monitor blood glucose and to continue to visit their primary care physician).[66]

Close follow-up, even using simple methods such as telephone calls, can be effective in identifying problems early and demonstrating the health-care team's commitment and concern for the patient.[67–69] Mail or telephone reminders about appointments also make follow-up easier because patients are less likely to forget their appointments.[70]

Technology-Based Adherence Aids

In the age of electronics and digitization, it sometimes seems that all the technology may get in the way of humanistic medical care. While this may be true in some regards, such as in the case of technological images and screens such as MRIs and

Table 7.2 Comparison of features in internet patient decision-support tools.

	Patient video interviews	Online community network	User-specific outcomes data	Access
FIMDM*	No	No	No	Web services for subscribers only
CHESS	Yes	Yes	No	Access limited to consortium member groups
NexCura	No	No	Yes	Free access through cobranded partner site; registration required
DIPEx	Yes	No[†]	No	Free on the Web
MayoClinic.com	Yes	No	No[‡]	Free on the Web

* Currently none of FIMDM's outcomes data and patient interviews are available on the Internet.
† DIPEx is currently redesigning and evaluating the concept of an online social support network.
‡ MayoClinic.com pilot project to tailor breast cancer adjuvant therapy data is in development.
J Med Internet Res. 2002 Oct–Dec; 4(2): e11.
Published online 2002 November 22. doi: 10.2196/jmir.4.2.e11.

CTs that depict the inside of the body,[71] technology can also play an important role in high quality medical care. Many patients report that their clinicians seem more familiar with their medical records when those records are computerized;[72] and many patients better understand their treatment through the use of digital tools.[35]

Some of the simplest technological interventions are aimed at improving patient adherence with innovations like special caps for medication bottles that record the last day and time the cap was removed. This type of tracking system has been shown to improve adherence rates by helping patients remember if and when they took their last dose of medication. In one study of hypertensive patients, those who were able to check and monitor their medication doses in this way achieved 95 percent adherence. Patients who had standard medication vials achieved only 78 percent adherence. In addition, patients with the timepiece caps experienced significant decreases in both their systolic and diastolic blood pressure, whereas those with standard vials had no change in their blood pressure from the baseline study measures. Combining the timepiece caps with home blood pressure testing devices and cards on which to keep records of their progress in controlling their hypertension resulted in a nearly 100 percent adherence rate for patients in this study, over a

12-week period.[73] This is particularly impressive given that these patients did not know they were being monitored for adherence and instead believed they were simply evaluating new materials and devices for people with high blood pressure.

Another adherence aid that uses electronic vial caps works differently but also quite effectively. Instead of recording and showing the date and time of the last dose so that patients can check themselves, these caps transmit to the health professional a record of each time the bottle is opened (and presumably medication is taken). The detailed record that results can be useful for clinicians as they discuss with their patients the ways in which they might improve their adherence.[74]

More sophisticated medication reminders, such as automated cell phone calls and PDA notifications are now being marketed, though their ability to foster adherence is not yet well established and more data on their effectiveness are needed.[75] A recent review of studies using electronic medication reminders for HIV patients revealed enhanced adherence in 4 of 8 studies, and only limited evidence of improved clinical outcomes.[76] Although the evidence that electronic reminders increase adherence is not robust, in none of the studies reviewed did the reminders *decrease* adherence. Further, patients uniformly reported satisfaction with the reminders regardless of whether other outcomes were measurably changed.[76]

One factor that may have influenced the results of this particular review is the complexity of adhering to antiretroviral therapy regimens. When the behavior required is less complicated (e.g., eye drops for glaucoma patients, daily asthma medications to help with breathing, oral contraceptive use), electronic reminders are more effective.[77–80]

Many websites are also available to help patients better adhere to their health-care regimens—most, however, focus on medication adherence. Some of these include the FDA website with information on safely using medications (www.fda. gov.cder/consumerinfo/ensuring_safe_use_all_resources.htm#brochures);   the LifeClinic site, which provides fitness and nutrition information as well as information on managing chronic health problems like diabetes, hypertension, and cholesterol (www.lifeclinic.com); and a clearinghouse-style website that provides links to commercial sites that market various adherence-improvement products (www.patientcompliance.net).

Many others are aimed at health professionals, however, to help them more effectively work with their patients who are trying to adhere. The American Heart Association's site, which also has a section for patients, provides a "compliance action program" for practitioners (www.americanheart.org); the National Council on Patient Information and Education's site has many useful resources to help improve communication with patients about appropriate medication use (www.talkaboutrx.org); and the United States Pharmacopeia has a library of 81 medicine descriptions, instructions, and warnings along with pictograms of each, which can be quite useful when working with patients who are low in health literacy or whose first language is not English (www.usp.org/audiences/consumers/pictograms). These resources can help patients and clinicians improve some of the skills that are so important to achieving medication adherence.

Table 7.3 Technology-based adherence aids

Electronic pill bottle cap that reminds patient
Electronic pill bottle cap that sends information to HCP when bottle is
    opened
Cell phone/text message reminder
PDA reminder
E-mail reminder

Digital Support Groups

Support groups and peer communities for people with shared health concerns
are not new, but the "virtual" or "digital" variety has only recently gained
popularity. Systematic evaluation of these virtual communities is difficult
because they are often embedded in a complex system of care delivery and
have seldom been subjected to rigorous empirical study methods. In addition,
they come in all types including online discussion groups and chat rooms,
newsgroups, e-mail lists, and voice bulletin board systems. It is likely that
such groups are more popular with individuals who have grown up with or
adapted to, electronic communication methods of various types; and this implies
that these groups may become increasingly popular and useful in the health-
care context.

One detailed review of the outcomes of various types of electronic peer
groups found little evidence that they improved health outcomes, but also did
not find any evidence that these groups posed any risk to participants.[81] One
study included in this review found that *participation* was significantly higher for
the virtual versus the face-to-face group[82] but another study found that virtual
groups were not as *effective* as face-to-face groups.[83] This suggests that perhaps
the ideal is to make both kinds of groups available so that patients might choose
the one that best fits their own needs and lifestyle. Certain aspects of the support
network, such as the sense of community, may be weaker in virtual groups but
their convenience might allow those who would be otherwise disinclined to
participate at all to engage in at least some form of supportive community
network. The authors of this review-style study emphasize that the absence of
evidence for the effectiveness of virtual communities doesn't mean that these
electronic groups are *not* useful; the types of studies that could better answer
this question still need to be conducted.

With regard to virtual groups, it is also worth mentioning the suggestion of
some critics that participation in online groups might stifle in-person social interactions or that the quality of such groups might lead to harm for participants.[84–86]
The fact that this review[81] found no such evidence is encouraging although, of
course, the absence of evident harm also does not mean that no risk is present.

Conclusion

This chapter underscores the importance of efficient use of precious time in medical visits. There are many strategies available to ensure that all-important discussions of health behavior change and adherence are not neglected. These strategies may include employing a team-oriented approach or using technology to share information between clinician and patient. Both health-care providers and patients may bring more tools to the visit when they utilize the technological resources that are available to them.

References

1. Center for Studying Health System Change. Community Tracking Study Physician Survey 2004–2005 [cited 2008 November 1]; Available from: http://CTSonline.s-3.com/psurvey.asp.
2. Crane JA. Patient comprehension of doctor-patient communication on discharge from the emergency department. J Emerg Med. 1997 Jan–Feb;15(1):1–7.
3. Roter DL, Hall JA. Studies of doctor-patient interaction. Annu Rev Public Health. 1989;10:163–80.
4. Bodenheimer T, Laing BY. The teamlet model of primary care. Ann Fam Med. 2007 Sep–Oct;5(5):457–61.
5. Baldwin DC. The role of interdisciplinary education and teamwork in primary care and health care reform. Rockville, MD: Health Resources and Services Administration, Bureau of Health Professions; 1994.
6. Bogden PE, Abbott RD, Williamson P, Onopa JK, Koontz LM. Comparing standard care with a physician and pharmacist team approach for uncontrolled hypertension. J Gen Intern Med. 1998 Nov;13(11):740–5.
7. Flood AB, Fremont AM, Jin K, Bott DM, Ding J, Parker RC, Jr. How do HMOs achieve savings? The effectiveness of one organization's strategies. Health Serv Res. 1998 Apr;33(1):79–99.
8. Grumbach K, Bodenheimer T. Can health care teams improve primary care practice? JAMA. 2004 Mar 10;291(10):1246–51.
9. Kottke TE, Brekke ML, Solberg LI. Making "time" for preventive services. Mayo Clin Proc. 1993 Aug;68(8):785–91.
10. Sommers LS, Marton KI, Barbaccia JC, Randolph J. Physician, nurse, and social worker collaboration in primary care for chronically ill seniors. Arch Intern Med. 2000 Jun 26; 160(12):1825–33.
11. Venning P, Durie A, Roland M, Roberts C, Leese B. Randomised controlled trial comparing cost effectiveness of general practitioners and nurse practitioners in primary care. BMJ. 2000 Apr 15;320(7241):1048–53.
12. Wagner EH. The role of patient care teams in chronic disease management. BMJ. 2000 Feb 26;320(7234):569–72.
13. Starfield B. Primary Care: Concept, Evaluation, and Policy. New York: Oxford University Press; 1992.
14. Wagner EH. Chronic disease management: what will it take to improve care for chronic illness? Eff Clin Pract. 1998 Aug–Sep;1(1):2–4.

15. Wagner EH, Austin BT, Von Korff M. Organizing care for patients with chronic illness. Milbank Q. 1996;74(4):511–44.
16. Campbell SM, Hann M, Hacker J, Burns C, Oliver D, Thapar A, Mead N, Safran DG, Roland MO. Identifying predictors of high quality care in English general practice: observational study. BMJ. 2001 Oct 6;323(7316):784–7.
17. Goni S. An analysis of the effectiveness of Spanish primary health care teams. Health Policy. 1999 Aug;48(2):107–17.
18. Safran DG. Defining the future of primary care: what can we learn from patients? Ann Intern Med. 2003 Feb 4;138(3):248–55.
19. Stevenson K, Baker R, Farooqi A, Sorrie R, Khunti K. Features of primary health care teams associated with successful quality improvement of diabetes care: a qualitative study. Fam Pract. 2001 Feb;18(1):21–6.
20. Vahey DC, Aiken LH, Sloane DM, Clarke SP, Vargas D. Nurse burnout and patient satisfaction. Med Care. 2004 Feb;42(2 Suppl):II57–66.
21. Donchin Y, Gopher D, Olin M, Badihi Y, Biesky M, Sprung CL, Pizov R, Cotev S. A look into the nature and causes of human errors in the intensive care unit. Crit Care Med. 1995 Feb;23(2):294–300.
22. Hadlow J, Pitts M. The understanding of common health terms by doctors, nurses, and patients. Soc Sci Med. 1991;32(2):193–6.
23. Cohen SG, Bailey DE. What makes teams work: group effectiveness research from the shop floor to the executive suite. Journal of Management. 1997;23(3):239–90.
24. Starfield B. Primary Care: Balancing Health Needs, Services, and Technology. New York: Oxford University Press; 1998.
25. Brown SA, Grimes DE. A meta-analysis of nurse practitioners and nurse midwives in primary care. Nursing Res. 1995 Nov–Dec;44(6):332–9.
26. Horrocks S, Anderson E, Salisbury C. Systematic review of whether nurse practitioners working in primary care can provide equivalent care to doctors. BMJ. 2002 Apr 6; 324(7341):819–23.
27. Lencioni PM. Make your values mean something. Harv Bus Rev. 2002 Jul;80(7):113–7, 26.
28. Haas LJ, Glazer K, Houchins J, Terry S. Improving the effectiveness of the medical visit: a brief visit-structuring workshop changes patients' perceptions of primary care visits. Patient Educ Couns. 2006 Sep;62(3):374–8.
29. DiMatteo MR, Reiter RC, Gambone JG. Enhancing medication adherence through communication and informed collaborative choice. Health Commun. 1994;6(4):253–65.
30. Baker LH, O'Connell D, Platt FW. "What else?" Setting the agenda for the clinical interview. Ann Intern Med. 2005 Nov 15;143(10):766–70.
31. Rodriguez HP, Anastario MP, Frankel RM, Odigie EG, Rogers WH, von Glahn T, Safran DG. Can teaching agenda-setting skills to physicians improve clinical interaction quality? A controlled intervention. BMC Medical Education. 2008;8:3.
32. Ball MJ, Lillis J. E-health: transforming the physician/patient relationship. Int J Med Inform. 2001 Apr;61(1):1–10.
33. Schneider SJ, Schwartz MD, Fast J. Computerized, telephone-based health promotion: I. Smoking cessation program. Computers in Human Behavior. 1995;11(1):135–48.
34. Turner CF, Ku L, Rogers SM, Lindberg LD, Pleck JH, Sonenstein FL. Adolescent sexual behavior, drug use, and violence: increased reporting with computer survey technology. Science. 1998 May 8, 1998;280(5365):867–73.

35. Noell J, Glasgow RE. Interactive technology applications for behavioral counseling: issues and opportunities for health care settings. Am J Prev Med. 1999 Nov;17(4):269–74.
36. Bates DW, Leape LL, Cullen DJ, Laird N, Petersen LA, Teich JM, Burdick E, Hickey M, Kleefield S, Shea B, Vander Vliet M, Seger DL. Effect of computerized physician order entry and a team intervention on prevention of serious medication errors. JAMA. 1998 Oct 21;280(15):1311–6.
37. Sproull L, Kiesler S. Connections: New Ways of Working in the Networked Organization. Cambridge, MA: MIT Press; 1991.
38. Spiro D, Heidrich F. Lay understanding of medical terminology. J Fam Pract. 1983 Aug;17(2):277–9.
39. Marshall PD. Bridging the terminology gap between health care professionals and patients with the Consumer Health Terminology (CHT). Proceedings of the Amer Medical Informatics Assn Symposium. 2000:1082.
40. Zeng QT, Tse T. Exploring and developing consumer health vocabularies. J Am Med Inform Assoc. 2006 Jan–Feb;13(1):24–9.
41. Zielstorff RD. Controlled vocabularies for consumer health. J Biomed Inform. 2003 Aug–Oct;36(4–5):326–33.
42. Centers for Disease Control and Prevention. Update: HIV counseling and testing using rapid tests—United States, 1995. MMWR Morb Mortal Wkly Rep. 1998;47(11):211–5.
43. Kunst H, Groot D, Latthe PM, Latthe M, Khan KS. Accuracy of information on apparently credible websites: survey of five common health topics. BMJ. 2002 Mar 9;324(7337):581–2.
44. Neuhauser L, Kreps G. Rethinking communication in the e-health era. J Health Psychol. 2003;8(1):7–23.
45. Tate DF, Wing RR, Winett RA. Using Internet technology to deliver a behavioral weight loss program. JAMA. 2001 Mar 7;285(9):1172–7.
46. Cassell MM, Jackson C, Cheuvront B. Health communication on the Internet: an effective channel for health behavior change? J Health Commun. 1998 Jan–Mar;3(1):71–9.
47. Kreps G. The role of interactive technology in cancer communications interventions: Targeting key audience members by tailoring messages. American Public Health Association Conference; Boston, MA. 2000.
48. Fotheringham MJ, Owies D, Leslie E, Owen N. Interactive health communication in preventive medicine: Internet-based strategies in teaching and research. Am J Prev Med. 2000 Aug;19(2):113–20.
49. Balas EA, Jaffrey F, Kuperman GJ, Boren SA, Brown GD, Pinciroli F, Mitchell JA. Electronic communication with patients. Evaluation of distance medicine technology. JAMA. 1997 Jul 9;278(2):152–9.
50. Krishna S, Balas EA, Spencer DC, Griffin JZ, Boren SA. Clinical trials of interactive computerized patient education: implications for family practice. J Fam Pract. 1997 Jul;45(1):25–33.
51. Lewis D. Computer-based approaches to patient education. J Am Med Inform Assoc. 1999;6:272–82.
52. Revere D, Dunbar PJ. Review of computer-generated outpatient health behavior interventions: clinical encounters "in absentia." J Am Med Inform Assoc. 2001 Jan–Feb;8(1):62–79.

53. Rimer BK, Halabi S, Sugg Skinner C, Kaplan EB, Crawford Y, Samsa GP, Strigo TS, Lipkus IM. The short-term impact of tailored mammography decision-making interventions. Patient Educ Couns. 2001 Jun;43(3):269–85.

54. Prochaska JJ, Zabinski MF, Calfas KJ, Sallis JF, Patrick K. PACE+: interactive communication technology for behavior change in clinical settings. Am J Prev Med. 2000 Aug;19(2):127–31.

55. Guendelman S, Meade K, Benson M, Chen YQ, Samuels S. Improving asthma outcomes and self-management behaviors of inner-city children: a randomized trial of the Health Buddy interactive device and an asthma diary. Arch Pediatr Adolesc Med. 2002 Feb;156(2):114–20.

56. Noffsinger EB, Scott JC. Understanding today's group-visit models. Group Practice Journal. 2000;48(2):46–8, 50, 2–4, 6–8.

57. Beck A, Scott J, Williams P, Robertson B, Jackson D, Gade G, Cowan P. A randomized trial of group outpatient visits for chronically ill older HMO members: the Cooperative Health Care Clinic. J Am Geriatr Soc. 1997 May;45(5):543–9.

58. Trento M, Passera P, Tomalino M, Bajardi M, Pomero F, Allione A, Vaccari P, Molinatti GM, Porta M. Group visits improve metabolic control in type 2 diabetes: a 2-year follow-\up. Diabetes Care. 2001 Jun;24(6):995–1000.

59. Butcher L. Shared decision-making aids improving, winning support among both patients & physicians for treatment choices. Oncology Times. 2008;30(10):23.

60. Kasper JF, Mulley AG, Wennberg JE. Developing shared decision-making programs to improve the quality of health care. Quality Review Bull. 1992;18(6):182.

61. Barry MJ. Health decision aids to facilitate shared decision making in office practice. Ann Intern Med. 2002 Jan 15;136(2):127–35.

62. Wilkins E, Lowery J, Hamill J. The impact of shared decision making in prostate specific antigen (PSA) screening. Med Decision Making. 1999;19:525.

63. Schwitzer G. A review of features in Internet consumer health decision-support tools. J Med Internet Res. 2002 Apr–Nov;4(2):E11.

64. Morgan MW, Deber RB, Llewellyn-Thomas HA, Gladstone P, Cusimano RJ, O'Rourke K, Tomlinson G, Detsky AS. Randomized, controlled trial of an interactive videodisc decision aid for patients with ischemic heart disease. J Gen Intern Med. 2000 Oct;15(10):685–93.

65. Murray E, Davis H, Tai SS, Coulter A, Gray A, Haines A. Randomised controlled trial of an interactive multimedia decision aid on hormone replacement therapy in primary care. BMJ (Clinical Research Ed). 2001 Sep 1;323(7311):490–3.

66. Aubert RE, Herman WH, Waters J, Moore W, Sutton D, Peterson BL, Bailey CM, Koplan JP. Nurse case management to improve glycemic control in diabetic patients in a health maintenance organization. A randomized, controlled trial. Ann Intern Med. 1998 Oct 15;129(8):605–12.

67. Maisiak R, Austin J, Heck L. Health outcomes of two telephone interventions for patients with rheumatoid arthritis or osteoarthritis. Arthritis Rheum. 1996 Aug;39(8):1391–9.

68. Von Korff M, Gruman J, Schaefer J, Curry SJ, Wagner EH. Collaborative management of chronic illness. Ann Intern Med. 1997 December 15, 1997;127(12):1097–102.

69. Wasson J, Gaudette C, Whaley F, Sauvigne A, Baribeau P, Welch HG. Telephone care as a substitute for routine clinic follow-up. JAMA. 1992 Apr 1;267(13):1788–93.

70. Macharia WM, Leon G, Rowe BH, Stephenson BJ, Haynes RB. An overview of interventions to improve compliance with appointment keeping for medical services. JAMA. 1992 Apr 1;267(13):1813–7.

71. Barnard A, Sandelowski M. Technology and humane nursing care: (ir)reconcilable or invented difference? J Adv Nurs. 2001 May;34(3):367–75.

72. Churgin PG. Computerized patient records: the patients' response. HMO Pract. 1995 Dec;9(4):182–5.

73. McKenney JM, Munroe WP, Wright JT, Jr. Impact of an electronic medication compliance aid on long-term blood pressure control. J Clin Pharmacol. 1992 Mar;32(3):277–83.

74. Rosen MI, Rigsby MO, Salahi JT, Ryan CE, Cramer JA. Electronic monitoring and counseling to improve medication adherence. Behavior Research and Therapy. 2003;42(4):409–22.

75. Sterns A, Collins, S. Transforming the personal digital assistant into a health-enhancing technology. Generations. 2004;28:54–6.

76. Wise J, Operario D. Use of electronic reminder devices to improve adherence to antiretroviral therapy: a systematic review. AIDS Patient Care and STDS. 2008 Jun;22(6):495–504.

77. Boden C, Sit A, Weinreb RN. Accuracy of an electronic monitoring and reminder device for use with travoprost eye drops. J Glaucoma. 2006 Feb;15(1):30–4.

78. Fish L, Lung CL. Adherence to asthma therapy. Ann Allergy Asthma Immunol. 2001 Jun;86(6 Suppl 1):24–30.

79. Fox MC, Creinin MD, Murthy AS, Harwood B, Reid LM. Feasibility study of the use of a daily electronic mail reminder to improve oral contraceptive compliance. Contraception. 2003 Nov;68(5):365–71.

80. Krueger KP, Felkey BG, Berger BA. Improving adherence and persistence: a review and assessment of interventions and description of steps toward a national adherence initiative. J Am Pharm Assoc. 2003 Nov–Dec;43(6):668–78; quiz 78–9.

81. Eysenbach G, Powell J, Englesakis M, Rizo C, Stern A. Health related virtual communities and electronic support groups: systematic review of the effects of online peer to peer interactions. BMJ. 2004 May 15;328(7449):1166.

82. Alemi F, Mosavel M, Stephens RC, Ghadiri A, Krishnaswamy J, Thakkar H. Electronic self-help and support groups. Med Care. 1996 Oct;34(10 Suppl):OS32–44.

83. Gary TL, Genkinger JM, Guallar E, Peyrot M, Brancati FL. Meta-analysis of randomized educational and behavioral interventions in type 2 diabetes. Diabetes Educ. 2003 May–Jun;29(3):488–501.

84. Culver JD, Gerr F, Frumkin H. Medical information on the Internet: a study of an electronic bulletin board. J Gen Intern Med. 1997 Aug;12(8):466–70.

85. Cummings JN, Butler B, Kraut r. The quality of online social relationships. Communications of the ACM. 2002;45(7):103–8.

86. Houghton AR, Wolstenholme CR, Hudson I. What questions do patients ask in a cardiology newsgroup and how reliable are the answers? Br J Cardiol. 2001;8:165–8.

8

Partnering for Adherence in the Healthcare System

If you don't know where you are going, any road will get you there.
—Lewis Carroll, English novelist

Nobody is perfect. Even if a person truly understands and is fully committed to a medical regimen, the regimen still may not be carried out successfully over time. Adherence can never be assumed, and every person is at risk of failing to carry out health-related plans.[1] Although the importance of patient adherence has been well recognized, and there has been an abundance of research on the subject, adherence rates have not changed dramatically in the past 30 years. Studies prior to 1980 showed, on average, about 63 percent adherence, while those in the decades since then estimate average adherence to be closer to 76 percent, which is an improvement but still reflects a failure rate of nearly one-fourth.[2]

Successful adherence is influenced by many factors, including disease type, the complexity of the regimen, patient resources, system-level barriers, the clinician-patient relationship itself,[2] and various cultural beliefs and experiences[3] (see Figure 8.1). Overall, about one-fourth of patients fail to follow their prescribed treatment regimens.[2, 4, 5] The preceding chapters have offered tips and strategies for informing, motivating, and encouraging health behavior change, and we proposed that health-care professionals could be optimistic about patients' abilities to successfully make and adhere to changes in their lives when the proper strategies are thoughtfully and carefully applied. Coming from this perspective, it may seem surprising that rates of nonadherence are so high. The idea that everyone is vulnerable to nonadherence may seem too pessimistic or exaggerated. We argue here, however, that it is not, and that increasing the likelihood of success requires frank recognition of the vulnerabilities and risk factors for nonadherence. Of course, it is important to keep in mind that there is no "typical" picture of the nonadherent patient.

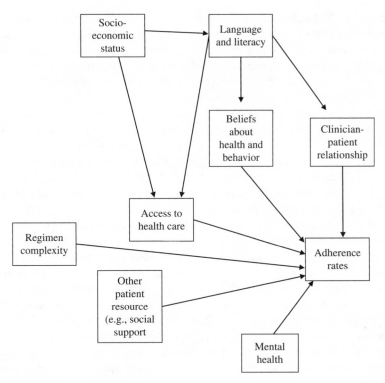

Figure 8.1 Influences on adherence.

Let us begin a closer examination of adherence by considering the following two scenarios. Abby is HIV positive, and although she still feels quite healthy, she has not been very good at keeping up with the complex medication regimen that her physician prescribed for her. So Abby recently began taking some newer medications with a simpler dosing schedule involving fewer pills taken less frequently. At first, she and her physician were both optimistic that, with this less demanding schedule, Abby would be able to take her medications as prescribed. Even with this new treatment approach, however, Abby has still not been as adherent as she needs to be. After only two months on the new regimen, her adherence rates fell to nearly as low as they were with her old program. Both she and the members of her health-care team now recognize that Abby's adherence depends not only on the prescription of a simpler regimen but also on other factors that must be clarified and dealt with concurrently.

Eric is also HIV positive. Like Abby he feels generally healthy, and he has recently switched to a relatively simple drug-dosing schedule. Unlike Abby, though, Eric's adherence *is* much improved after only two months on his new treatment plan. Not surprisingly, there were a few rough spots in the first couple of weeks as Eric adjusted to the new schedule and worked to improve his medication consistency (something he'd pretty much given up on with his previous, very complex drug regimen). These initial failures didn't surprise or discourage him, though. He and his doctor discussed the challenges he encountered, most of which had been anticipated even before he began his new treatment. Eric had been assigned a health educator to follow up with him periodically and whom he can call any time with questions. Eric also received some inexpensive record-keeping materials, including a medication diary to help him track his own progress with the new drugs. Simplifying Eric's medical regimen certainly helped him to become more adherent, but his own recognition that it would still take a lot of effort was also critical. It was essential to put into place the appropriate mechanisms to enhance Eric's efforts toward adherence success.

These two scenarios, of Abby and Eric, illustrate that even two people with the same illness and similar regimens may have different barriers to adherence; understanding the challenges for each individual person is a key goal for a clinician. In this chapter, we pinpoint many of these specific barriers to successful adherence at both the individual and the system level, and we identify various possible strategies for improving adherence, emphasizing that these will be most apparent and their implementation most feasible when patients and clinicians actively work together as partners in the patient's care. We also remind readers of the *information-motivation-strategy model* and encourage attention to possible barriers and tools that occur within each of these three broad categories. Many of these barriers are summarized in Table 8.1, which also provides examples of how clinicians might partner with patients to improve adherence.

Table 8.1 Common barriers to adherence and strategies for addressing them.

Barrier	Strategy
Number of medications	Reduce number of medications by using combination drugs, timed-release pills, etc. Make sure that the patient really needs all prescribed medications.
Complexity of the regimen (medication and/or lifestyle)	Reduce complexity, if possible. Integrate aspects of regimen into patient's schedule of daily life (e.g., encourage patient to take time to do recommended stretches while coffee is brewing; provide recipes for more healthy versions of favorite dishes). Link health behaviors to already existing behaviors (e.g., keep medications next to coffee maker).

Table 8.1 (Continued)

Perceived side effects (expected and experienced)	Discuss side effects with patients, being sure that they accurately understand the likelihood of such effects. If side effects are experienced, make adjustments to regimen to alleviate these, if possible (e.g., switch medications, prescribe additional medication to reduce side effects). Be sure patients understand cofactors (such as dietary restrictions) that might affect their experienced side effects if not followed accurately.
Reason for following regimen is not clear, or outcomes are distant	Discuss with patients the links between adherence and outcomes (and outcomes associated with nonadherence); reinforce that changes do not happen immediately; help them to have realistic expectations about the outcomes associated with adherence.
Lack of financial resources	Provide help with filing insurance claims and identifying resources for assistance; help patients identify less costly alternatives (e.g., walking trails near home instead of purchasing a gym membership); encourage cost-saving strategies such as ordering medications by mail.
Hectic schedule, no time	Emphasize with patients the importance of finding time; work with patients to identify ways that the regimen can be integrated with personal schedule.
Hectic schedule, forgetting	Encourage use of reminders such as pill boxes, PDA or text message prompts, medication calendars, etc. Supply reminders to patient if possible.
Lack of social support	Encourage patients to request support from family members and friends; initiate contact with family members and request their support in specific ways, if appropriate; encourage patient to join support group, and provide information about such groups.
Low health literacy, lack of understanding about what should be done	Take time to explain clearly to patient, avoiding jargon and checking frequently for patient understanding. Discuss with patient in a relaxing, quiet environment that is free of distractions. Provide patient with access to educational materials (interactive, if possible). Provide written / visual materials (e.g., pictures) to aid understanding and memory.

(Continued)

Table 8.1 (Continued)

Barrier	Strategy
Low self-efficacy for health behavior	Encourage greater self-efficacy using the strategies of personal experience, vicarious experience, and verbal persuasion.
Lack of positive reinforcement for following regimen	Praise patient successes and reinforce their relevance to overall health goals; encourage family members to positively reinforce patient; help patient set up contingency plans to self-monitor and reward adherence to plan.
Lack of access to needed facilities or treatments	Help patient identify community resources or assistance programs.
Interference of other problems (e.g., being unable to perform recommended exercises because of another health issue)	Work with patient to find alternative ways of carrying out desired behavior; discuss ways to minimize interference.

Simplicity and Quality of Life

For both Abby and Eric, the complexity of the treatment process created one barrier to successful adherence; these two patients are not alone in experiencing this challenge. Regimen complexity is one of the best-known barriers to adherence,[2, 4, 6, 7] and when directives involve lifestyle changes (such as in exercise patterns and diet) the challenges may be even greater than they are with medication alone. Changing one's lifestyle can be quite difficult. As we described in Chapter 4, eating, exercise, sleep and other health behaviors become ingrained in our lives as habits, and breaking an established habit can be even more difficult than trying to simply form a new one, such as when learning to regularly take three pills every day or to make an evening walk habitual. Stopping a behavior that serves a function and has been reinforced over a long period of time can be extremely challenging, yet it is often the case that treatment regimens involve stopping certain behaviors while at the same time starting new ones.

How can regimens be simplified? When medication is involved, one way to simplify is to reduce the pill burden. One study found that among HIV patients taking antiretroviral medications, the most frequent reason for missing their doses was that they forgot (66%), followed by their being away from home (57%), being busy with other things (53%), and having a change in daily routine (51%).[8] Another study, this one a quantitative review of HIV patients' virological responses to HAART (highly active antiretroviral therapy), found that the best predictor of achieving virus levels that were undetectable (i.e., HIV-RNA plasma levels) was a lower daily pill burden. Appropriate adherence is easier to achieve when patients need to take few pills per day than when they are required to take many,[9] and the best adherence rates are associated with once-daily dosing as compared to twice- or thrice-daily dosing.[10, 11] Some conditions have even less frequent dosing, such as monthly or even annually (e.g., for postmenopausal osteoporosis).

Complex medication regimens are not only difficult to carry out accurately, they can also *feel* overwhelming to patients. One common reason that patients give for discontinuing HAART (not just missing doses!) is that they have too many pills to take.[9, 12] Thus, decreasing the dosing frequency not only makes the regimens more manageable, it also helps them *feel* manageable which, in turn, encourages patients to continue to put forth the effort necessary to adhere. Of course, it may not always be possible to bring a complex medication regimen down to one or even two or three pills per day. Time-release or combination tablets (that combine several drugs into a single pill) can sometimes help to decrease the total number of pills that must be taken per day, however. Combination drugs for HIV, for example, have demonstrated efficacy in helping to manage difficult treatment regimens,[13] and combination antihypertensive drugs are also effective.[14]

Another step toward enhancing medication adherence involves clearly explaining to patients the dietary and other lifestyle requirements that may accompany their dosing regimens. Research shows that when the regimen is complex (such as involving the requirement that a pill cannot be taken with dairy products, or that it must be taken on an empty stomach, or that it must be taken exactly every four hours), adherence rates are often dramatically lower than when adherence requirements are more simple.[15, 16] The necessity of following specific directives and regimen requirements, and the reasoning behind them, must be made clear to patients lest they ignore them if they become inconvenient, thus reducing the effectiveness of the medications or even creating new problems.

The side effects of many regimens, particularly those involving medication, also help determine whether a patient is likely to adhere to a protocol.[17] Although it is certainly desirable to choose medications that have few (or no) side effects, this isn't always possible. If unpleasant side effects are likely to occur, anticipating them and identifying tools that will enable the individual to manage them can be crucial.[7] Patients may, for example, be able to take another medication to alleviate an unpleasant side effect, or changes in routine might be made to minimize their intrusiveness.

A strong social support network is another tool that can be very helpful in the self-management process.[2, 18, 19] In Chapter 2 we noted the importance of social norms and expectations for motivating a desire to change, and in Chapter 4 we saw evidence of the importance of social networks for helping monitor and regulate behavior. Here, we again see the importance of social support, as we recognize that members of one's support network may be able to provide various forms of support for adherence, such as instrumental, informational, and emotional support.[20]

Instrumental support is concrete in nature and would include things like running errands for your grandmother if her medications cause her to be unable to drive, reminding your spouse to take his or her pills, or taking notes for a friend who has to miss class once per month in order to keep an important recurring medical appointment. *Informational support* involves sharing of information. Examples include giving your favorite low-sodium recipes to your aunt who is struggling with her new, and very bland, low-sodium diet or showing your coworker a convenient walking trail you've found near the office when he complains that he can't find time to walk as his physician has recommended. *Emotional support* is probably what most people think of when they hear the term "social support." It involves providing a listening ear and letting another person know that you care for them, acknowledging their struggles, and empathizing with them. Being emotionally supportive requires listening to the struggling individual's story, but will likely also involve encouraging and supportive statements such as "I admire the way you're managing these challenges" or "Anyone would feel discouraged after a day like that—don't give up, though." Depending on the nature of an individual's challenges, various combinations of these forms of social support may be needed. Being able to rely on friends and family for support can do a great deal to help a person succeed in reaching their adherence goals.

Eric, whom we considered earlier, not only anticipated with his health-care team some of the challenges of his new regimen, he also worked with those in his social circle to help him overcome these challenges. He was also able to rely on his partner, his best friend, and his HIV-support group for emotional support. Members of his HIV group offered lots of helpful recommendations for coping with challenges at work and with some of the physical symptoms he was facing. His best friend helped by running errands when Eric was feeling particularly tired, and his partner provided frequent reminders about the new medication schedule. These social supports facilitated Eric's adherence to his new regimen.

Unfortunately, Abby did not share the kinds of resources Eric had. Although perhaps not purposely, Abby's best friend was insensitive to her dietary and alcohol restrictions and often encouraged her to "try just a little" of something she was supposed to avoid. Abby frequently stayed out late socializing with friends, missing her support group meetings and compromising the sleep that her physician had told her was very important to her health. Because her time with friends was very important to her, she told herself that the fatigue she felt was due to the new medications, and several times when she was feeling especially tired she simply decided not to take them. In addition, some evenings when she came home late at night, she realized she had missed a medication dose, and depending on the timing would skip it altogether or would double up on the dose (though she wasn't sure she was supposed to do this). She didn't consult her doctor about the difficulties she was having, thinking she would just "wait and see."

Both Eric and Abby could have benefited from a simplified medication regimen, but only one of them did. Perhaps Abby, too, could have enjoyed more success if she had taken a more active role in her own treatment decisions; sharing the challenges she was experiencing would have allowed her health-care team the opportunity to work with her to create environments that were more conducive to success (including improving her social support system).

Patient-Centered Interventions

Earlier, we discussed several elements that make nonadherence more likely. But in some cases, a lack of understanding or a complex set of requirements is not the cause of the patient's "failure." Instead, nonadherence represents the individual's desire to maintain a sense of personal identity, control, and quality of life.[21–23] It is important for the clinician to understand such reasoning and accept and work with the patient's individual perspective. Taking medications or following special dietary guidelines, for example, might identify the patient to others as "different" and make the patient feel stigmatized. While sometimes Abby forgot to take her medications, there were other times when she remembered but decided to wait to take them later because she didn't want to take pills in front of her friends or coworkers.

Individuals also may resist feeling dependent on their medical care team, on drugs themselves, or on family members. When the health issue is one that develops slowly over time or may lead to a negative outcome far in the future (e.g., hypertension), there are few obvious and immediate repercussions associated with nonadherence. Thus, the present rewards associated with normalizing and "fitting in" with everyone else may take priority over long-term outcomes of health and disease management.[24, 25] The sense of belonging or feelings of independence and autonomy may seem more important at the moment than what can be expected years later in life if target health behaviors are compromised.

Reasoned or intentional nonadherence can often be tackled with a patient-centered approach. Regimens need to be devised that make sense to the patient and fit in with his or her own lifestyle, goals, past experiences and present unique situation. With real buy-in on the part of the patient, adherence becomes more likely and patient outcomes are likely to be improved.[26, 27] A patient-centered approach also includes a continuing dialogue, working with the patient throughout the illness experience, and making adaptations to the regimen as necessary over time.

How can patients be made the center of the treatment approach? By identifying what is important to patients and taking patient values and priorities into account during decision-making, the treatment becomes centered on the patient as a person (i.e., tailored treatment), instead of on the disease or the priorities of the medical staff. Such patient-centered care includes the following: a focus on how illness affects the patient, a holistic approach, sharing of perspectives on illness management, attention to promoting good health, and attention to improving the relationship.[28]

Table 8.2 Patient-centered versus traditional care.

Patient-centered	Traditional
Focus on how illness affects all aspects of the patient's life	Focus on how illness affects the patient physically
Holistic approach	Biomedical, focused approach
Shared decision-making regarding illness management	Health-care professional makes decisions and prescribes them to the patient
Promotion of good health, including psychosocial aspects	Focus on curing illness
Focus on improving the relationship	Focus on improving the patient's physical health only
Patient and clinician as experts, working together	Health-care professional as expert
Encourages patient autonomy, fosters self-management skills	Encourages patient to follow directives accurately

The patient-centered approach also emphasizes the patient's role as expert. Patients know what their symptoms mean to them; they experience health and illness within the context of their daily lives. Practitioners must ask questions and actively *listen* in order to gain understanding of the patient's viewpoint (see Chapter 6 regarding open-ended questions and other details of communication between patients and clinicians).

Patient-centeredness also involves increasing patient autonomy and supporting the patient's ability to effectively self-manage her or his condition, especially with regard to preventive health behaviors and chronic illnesses. Patient education has traditionally focused on teaching specific skills and increasing knowledge, but self-management emphasizes problem-solving and self-efficacy[29] thus providing a nice complement to the standard approaches. The self-management approach recognizes that patients indeed do manage their own behaviors, making countless health-related decisions every day.[30] Effective training involves paying attention to how patients carry out their self-management and to how well they are able to achieve their health goals, helping them to modify their techniques when necessary.

Patient-defined action plans with short-range goals play a major role in self-management. For example, a patient might make a commitment to go for a walk every day for the next two weeks, or to take medication every day for the next week. Patient-defined action plans are similar to "New Year's resolutions" but they involve distinct and proximal endpoints only one to a few weeks ahead.[31] Because they are chosen by patients to be realistic and achievable, they are more likely to be carried out than are plans not chosen by patients.

After succeeding, the patient develops a sense of self-efficacy and is then more likely to adopt another (perhaps slightly more ambitious) short-term goal. The patient's role here is crucial, of course. Only the patient knows what is feasible for him or her, and if the patient's confidence in her or his ability to complete the task is not at least a 7 (on a 0–10 scale) the goal should be modified so that the patient feels the goal is achievable.[29] Bringing the patient into the equation as a self-manager is much more effective than simply having the patient "carry out the doctor's orders," for two reasons.[29] First, it is more economical for a patient to self-manage; second, improved patient outcomes result when a patient self-manages.

Encouraging Self-Efficacy

In Chapter 2 we introduced the concept of self-efficacy. We highlighted how important it is in influencing an individual's adoption and pursuit of goal-oriented behaviors;[32–34] and we examined the factors that enhance one's sense of self-efficacy.[35] We noted that professionals who partner with patients to manage health are in a unique position to help patients expand their own beliefs about personal competence and ability.

Because verbal encouragement tends to be easy, it is the most commonly used method for promoting self-efficacy. Verbal encouragement, however, is less effective for an individual than having him or her experience (or observe) success. Further, the power of verbal encouragement tends to be diluted by overuse. The novelty wears off and the message becomes so repetitive that it is easy to ignore.

Thus, in conjunction with the verbal encouragement that is easy to provide, health-care personnel should actively seek to help their patients identify role models for success in their own lives. Health professionals might even choose to provide examples of similar patients (without any personally identifying information, of course!) whose stories offer the patient vicarious experiences. As the relationship develops and the clinician comes to better know the patient and her or his background, identifying these models with the patient becomes easier. Also, helping patients to connect with resources such as support groups, through which they can observe the successes of others, can be effective in increasing patients' vicarious experiences.

Creating an environment in which patients can attain and experience success for themselves may be one of the clinician's most vital roles and requires the most collaboration between clinician and patient. Outcomes will be best if the relationship is strong and comfortable so that the patient can freely describe his or her anticipated stumbling blocks and barriers. Outcomes will also be best if the patient feels comfortable questioning aspects of the health recommendations and responds to a little social pressure to carry out the jointly agreed-upon course of action. In conjunction with the patient, the clinician can encourage adoption of a sequence of health-related goals that are short-term and small enough that success for each is very likely. These successes foster the sense of self-efficacy that is so important to adopting even more ambitious goals and effectively carrying them out. Table 8.3 provides some examples of behaviors along with ways each technique for increasing self-efficacy might be used.

Table 8.3 Increasing adherence by fostering self-efficacy using three strategies.

Target behavior	Verbal persuasion	Vicarious experience	Personal experience
Self-monitor blood glucose at home on a regular basis; patient is squeamish.	"It's really not hard once you get used to it. You can do this."	Have patient watch several others use simple devices to obtain blood and take glucose reading.	First have someone else do the prick for blood and have patient get reading; then have patient do a supervised prick and reading.
Walk one to two miles each day; patient feels like a mile is beyond his ability.	"Just walk slowly and take your time. I have confidence that you *can* walk a mile!"	Allow patient to discuss in support group with others who have been successful in walking this distance daily.	Devise plan with patient whereby he walks a much smaller distance the first day and then slowly increases over time.
Eating healthfully; patient says she has little willpower and can't make "healthy versions" that taste good.	"You just have to be strong. I have faith in you. You can do it."	Help patient to identify people in her life who do eat healthfully and encourage role modeling after those individuals.	Have patient enroll in cooking class where she can successfully make tasty dishes. Devise plan with patient where one healthy choice is consciously made per day (gradually increasing).
Managing stress; patient doesn't believe he can learn to relax.	"I think this will really be something you can achieve. I know you're going to be successful."	Have the patient view videotapes or DVDs in which similar others describe their successes in learning to relax. If possible, have patient interact with people who are already using the skills the patient hopes to learn.	Help patient identify other times when he's taken on difficult tasks and been successful; find similarities in what's required and build on these. Devise plan where small gains are made in the ability to relax, building over time.

Multifaceted Interventions to Improve Adherence

We have noted that particularly when regimens are patient-centered and as simple as possible, they are more likely to succeed. Inasmuch as simple treatment or health behavior change regimens are desirable, however, the improvement of patient adherence requires multifaceted approaches. Changing behavior and helping patients to adhere requires interventions that are broad in terms of their implementation. Two reviews have noted that comprehensive interventions are more effective than those that focus on any single adherence barrier. Interventions are most effective when they combine different strategies and target cognitive, behavioral, and affective elements of the patients' experience.[36, 37] For example, a nicotine patch may indeed help a smoker to quit smoking. But a smoker who not only has a prescription for nicotine patches but also has joined a smoking cessation support group, has completed a behavioral contract, and will receive a health insurance discount after completing six smoke-free months is more likely to be successful than someone who relies on nothing more than nicotine patches and willpower.

And, when these interventions are coordinated among members of the health-care delivery team[38–40] and tailored to the individual, results are also improved.[37] To illustrate, let's consider the differences between Inda and Miriam. Both are trying to quit smoking, and both are fortunate enough to have more than just a nicotine patch to help them. Inda's smoking cessation plan is highly individualized and integrated. Each person she interacts with regarding her health—physician, nurse educator, and physical therapist (she is also rehabilitating from a broken ankle)—encourage her efforts to stop smoking and inquire about her progress. Even the office receptionist, with whom she has talked about her desire to quit, asks her how it's going! Her step-down plan has been carefully worked out with her nurse educator, taking into account several upcoming events where many smokers are likely to be present. She's had a family meeting during which she was able to garner specific elements of support from several key family members, and she's signed a behavioral contract in their presence. After two weeks, Inda has already gone from nearly a pack of cigarettes per day down to only three or four. She's on track and feeling motivated.

Miriam's plan has some of the same elements as Inda's. She has received formal commitments of help from family members; she has a step-down plan that was provided to her by a health educator; and she's signed a behavioral contract. She didn't have much input into the particulars of the step-down plan, though, and she hasn't really figured out a way to manage her at-work smoking effectively. Miriam usually succumbs to temptation when her office mates congregate on the patio to smoke. She intends to talk to her health educator about the difficulties she's having, but she hasn't gotten around to it yet. Although she has all the same information that Inda has about the risks of smoking and ways to stop, only her health educator discusses smoking with her. Miriam's primary care doctor mentions it only in passing and seems more concerned with whether she is taking her antihypertensive medications regularly. Thus, Miriam's progress toward becoming smoke-free has stalled several times, and in four months she hasn't even cut her cigarette consumption in half. Despite the fact that she's not meeting her goals, she feels okay about her progress since her physician doesn't seem worried about it.

These examples, and the research on which they are based, highlight the importance of personalizing interventions as noted in Chapter 4. They emphasize the importance of information and strategy synchronization across the care delivery experience (such as with a well-coordinated health-care team, discussed in Chapter 7). Thus, although it is important to make everything as simple as possible for the patient, the extra effort that is required of health professionals in order to implement a more multifaceted intervention is indeed worthwhile, because it results in better adherence outcomes for patients.

Partnering and Barriers within Health-Care Systems

Coordination of multifaceted interventions to improve adherence or other health behaviors is both more effective and more challenging than the "piecemeal" approach that often occurs in patient care (the embedded nature of multifaceted issues is illustrated in Figure 8.2). Staff-model HMOs may have some advantage

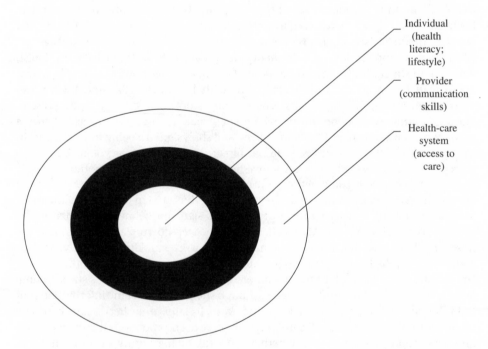

Individual
(health
literacy;
lifestyle)

Provider
(communication
skills)

Health-care
system
(access to
care)

Figure 8.2 Embedded nature of barriers to adherence within multifaceted interventions.

here because they already employ some elements of a team approach such as ease of access to patient records across specialties and the possibility for patients to have various appointments, trainings, or group interactions at a single location. Building effective partnerships may be more difficult within a managed care system that is spread out geographically, as well as for those who remain within the rapidly shrinking fee-for-service system.[41]

Patients do notice deficiencies in the coordination of their medical services, reporting that primary care, with a few notable exceptions, generally lacks a "whole-person" orientation with an emphasis on provider-patient partnerships, and on integration of care.[42] Some studies actually suggest that this trend is worsening and that patient care is becoming more and more fragmented.[41,43,44] This fragmentation, in turn, affects patients' ability to feel connected with their health-care providers even in cases where there is some continuity of care.[42] And, although there is evidence that many HMOs do focus on health behaviors such as preventive screening and preventive health behavior counseling,[45] patients often come to view their primary care physicians as gatekeepers to specialty services rather than as true partners in care.[46] Thus, despite the potential advantage with regard to teamwork that comes with a managed care system, it is not clear that a high level of integration always occurs.[44,47,48]

Whatever the model of health-care delivery, patients who are allowed to exercise more control, both with regard to choosing their primary care providers and to participating in their own care, experience more positive outcomes.[46,49,50] Their active role allows them to better navigate the health-care system and to overcome barriers (as well as enjoy benefits) at all of its levels, not just the personal level.

There is little doubt that there is a financial benefit to keeping people as healthy as possible. The most successful health-care organizations are those that effectively promote preventive health behaviors. Traditionally, medical care has tended to focus on secondary and tertiary levels of care (that is, care aimed at reducing risks or alleviating existing problems) rather than on primary prevention (care aimed at maintaining current good health and reducing *potential* risks).[51,52] But, with health-care dollars shrinking, more emphasis than ever needs to be placed on promoting health behavior change and enhancing patient adherence to recommended treatments. This best takes place within a patient-centered, collaborative care model.

Access to care

Many of the barriers to adherence that we have discussed in this book are unique to individuals, rooted in their own past experiences, cultural norms, and personal values. Health-care systems can coordinate the care that they deliver in order to best help patients overcome these barriers, but other barriers are presented by the system itself. Access to medical care is one of the system-level barriers that, as a social problem, continues to grow.

At the time of this writing, about 47 million people are without health insurance; millions more are underinsured, and cannot afford all of the care that they need. The Institute of Medicine has proposed six areas for care improvement in the twenty-first century[53] (safety, effectiveness, patient-centeredness, timeliness, efficiency, and equitability) yet access-related problems such as availability/affordability of care, appropriateness of care, care that meets patients' preferences, having a usual source of care, and timely delivery of care all challenge these six aims.[54] There are serious disparities in availability of care, as well, with minority patients and those with lower income having less access and as a result, poorer health.[55–57]

Having a usual source of care is important because patients who see the same physician regularly are more likely to have visits focused on prevention of future health problems.[58, 59] Having a usual physician does not guarantee patient health behaviors such as exercising or quitting smoking[59] but it does increase the opportunity for patients and doctors to discuss issues such as these and work toward health behavior change. Having a regular, integrated health-care *team* makes it even more likely that patients will be able to access the kind of help that they need at the time it will do them the most good.

Even if a patient has adequate health insurance or a good health management plan, the ability to receive timely care is sometimes problematic. For example, if a patient has a nonemergency medical issue but cannot miss work without penalty, it may be difficult to obtain the care that she or he is paying for. Timeliness of care can be compromised when a patient must make several preliminary visits before receiving a referral to a specialist. The patient might dread the length of this process and therefore delay seeking care.

When access to care that meets a patient's needs is limited, some health-care opportunities remain underused while others, such as emergency rooms, become overused.[54, 60, 61] Besides the incredible expense and overcrowding of emergency departments, the use of emergency care can create a cascade of problems throughout the system itself. Alleviation of presenting symptoms becomes the primary concern, and long-term planning and prevention become less central. This leads, in turn, to higher rates of acute symptoms and seeking of care at facilities designed for treating acute cases instead of preventing these problems from occurring in the first place.[62]

What Can Health Professionals Do?

In the absence of system-level change, individual health professionals can take steps to address issues of access to care. Health-care providers can offer their patients information, guidance, and programs to manage their own health conditions more autonomously. Health professionals may be able to have medical visits with patients in more varied ways. For example, they might schedule telephone appointments, confer with patients via e-mail, or create office visits in an "advanced access" format where patients don't have to wait long to be seen. Physicians might also staff mobile clinics,[54] work with other team members, and adopt some of the technologies as described in Chapter 7 to deliver care in the most efficient way possible.

Insurance status is another factor that is heavily influenced by systems and which influences health care at the individual level. Patients with insurance coverage are more likely to receive preventive health services, and they are particularly likely to receive preventive care if they have both insurance and a regular care provider.[58] Insured patients also tend to adhere to medication regimens more effectively because cost is less likely to be a barrier to their following through with treatment recommendations.[63] This is one area where patients with certain network-style health-care providers (such as those covered by the Veterans Health Administration) experience some advantage; they are less likely to cite monetary reasons for failing to take medications even when compared to those with private insurance.[63]

Each system of care and reimbursement has its own idiosyncrasies and thus each patient-clinician pair will need to work together creatively, and with a clear understanding of the issues presented by the system they are dealing with, in order to reach the best solutions for individual patients.

This chapter focuses on the importance of partnership between health-care professionals and patients, an issue which has been a common theme throughout this book. The goal of partnership is to work with patients to help them address their barriers to adherence and behavior change and to enable them to be active members of their own health-care teams. This requires an understanding of factors unique to each individual patient. Recognizing the various forms and degrees of challenge a patient might be encountering is also key, along with acknowledging that a patient is not solely to blame when she or he is nonadherent. The larger context of the health-care system in which the patient functions also plays an important role. Finally, in understanding these potential barriers, it is also important to keep in mind the simple three-factor model: information-motivation-strategy. Determining what patients know, what motivates them, and what their resources are is a simple and effective way to partner and communicate with patients about their health behaviors and adherence.

Keeping in mind the simple information-motivation-strategy formula—that people do only what they *understand*, what they *want* to do, and what they are *able* to do—and the many behavioral interventions suggested in this book, the dedicated health professional will be well equipped to educate, motivate, and assist patients toward better health behaviors and ultimately better health outcomes.

References

1. Porter AM. Drug defaulting in a general practice. Br Med J. 1969 Jan 25;1(5638):218–22.
2. DiMatteo MR. Variations in patients' adherence to medical recommendations: a quantitative review of 50 years of research. Med Care. 2004 Mar;42(3):200–9.
3. Carter S, Taylor D, Levenson R. A question of choice: Compliance in medicine taking. A preliminary review. Medicines Partnership; 2003.
4. Atreja A, Bellam N, Levy SR. Strategies to enhance patient adherence: making it simple. MedGenMed. 2005;7(1):4.
5. Dunbar-Jacob J, Burke LE, Pyczynski S. Clinical assessment and management of adherence to medical regimens. In: Nicassio PM, Smith TW, editors. Managing Chronic Illness: A Biopsychosocial Perspective. Washington, DC: American Psychological Association; 1995. p. 313–49.
6. Morningstar BA, Sketris IS, Kephart GC, Sclar DA. Variation in pharmacy prescription refill adherence measures by type of oral antihyperglycaemic drug therapy in seniors in Nova Scotia, Canada. J Clin Pharm Ther. 2002 Jun;27(3):213–20.
7. Trotta MP, Ammassari A, Melzi S, Zaccarelli M, Ladisa N, Sighinolfi L, Mura MS, d'Arminio Monforte A, Antinori A. Treatment-related factors and highly active antiretroviral therapy adherence. J Acquir Immune Defic Syndr. 2002 Dec 15;31 Suppl 3:S128–31.
8. Bartlett JA. Addressing the challenges of adherence. J Acquir Immune Defic Syndr. 2002 Feb 1;29 Suppl 1:S2–10.
9. Bartlett JA, DeMasi R, Quinn J, Moxham C, Rousseau F. Overview of the effectiveness of triple combination therapy in antiretroviral-naive HIV-1 infected adults. AIDS. 2001 Jul 27;15(11):1369–77.
10. Claxton AJ, Cramer J, Pierce C. A systematic review of the associations between dose regimens and medication compliance. Clin Ther. 2001 Aug;23(8):1296–310.
11. Eldred LJ, Wu AW, Chaisson RE, Moore RD. Adherence to antiretroviral and pneumocystis prophylaxis in HIV disease. J Acquir Immune Defic Syndr Hum Retrovirol. 1998 Jun 1;18(2):117–25.
12. Chesney MA, Ickovics JR, Chambers DB, Gifford AL, Neidig J, Zwickl B, Wu AW. Self-reported adherence to antiretroviral medications among participants in HIV clinical trials: the AACTG adherence instruments. Patient Care Committee & Adherence Working Group of the Outcomes Committee of the Adult AIDS Clinical Trials Group (AACTG). AIDS Care. 2000 Jun;12(3):255–66.
13. Eron JJ, Yetzer ES, Ruane PJ, Becker S, Sawyer GA, Fisher RL, Tolson JM, Shaefer MS. Efficacy, safety, and adherence with a twice-daily combination lamivudine/zidovudine tablet formulation, plus a protease inhibitor, in HIV infection. AIDS. 2000 Apr 14;14(6):671–81.
14. Skolnik NS, Beck JD, Clark M. Combination antihypertensive drugs: recommendations for use. Am Fam Physician. 2000 May 15;61(10):3049–56.
15. Nieuwkerk PT, Sprangers MA, Burger DM, Hoetelmans RM, Hugen PW, Danner SA, van Der Ende ME, Schneider MM, Schrey G, Meenhorst PL, Sprenger HG, Kauffmann RH, Jambroes M, Chesney MA, de Wolf F, Lange JM. Limited patient adherence to highly active antiretroviral therapy for HIV-1 infection in an observational cohort study. Arch Intern Med. 2001 Sep 10;161(16):1962–8.

16. Stone VE, Hogan JW, Schuman P, Rompalo AM, Howard AA, Korkontzelou C, Smith DK. Antiretroviral regimen complexity, self-reported adherence, and HIV patients' understanding of their regimens: survey of women in the HER study. J Acquir Immune Defic Syndr. 2001 Oct 1;28(2):124–31.
17. Ammassari A, Murri R, Pezzotti P, Trotta MP, Ravasio L, De Longis P, Lo Caputo S, Narciso P, Pauluzzi S, Carosi G, Nappa S, Piano P, Izzo CM, Lichtner M, Rezza G, Monforte A, Ippolito G, d'Arminio Moroni M, Wu AW, Antinori A. Self-reported symptoms and medication side effects influence adherence to highly active antiretroviral therapy in persons with HIV infection. J Acquir Immune Defic Syndr. 2001 Dec 15;28(5):445–9.
18. Cameron C. Patient compliance: recognition of factors involved and suggestions for promoting compliance with therapeutic regimens. J Adv Nurs. 1996 Aug;24(2):244–50.
19. Catz SL, Kelly JA, Bogart LM, Benotsch EG, McAuliffe TL. Patterns, correlates, and barriers to medication adherence among persons prescribed new treatments for HIV disease. Health Psychology: Official Journal of the Division of Health Psychology, American Psychological Association. 2000 Mar;19(2):124–33.
20. Uchino BN, Cacioppo JT, Kiecolt-Glaser JK. The relationship between social support and physiological processes: a review with emphasis on underlying mechanisms and implications for health. Psychological Bulletin. 1996 May;119(3):488–531.
21. Conrad P. The meaning of medications: another look at compliance. Soc Sci Med. 1985;20(1):29–37.
22. Lambert BL, Street RL, Cegala DJ, Smith DH, Kurtz S, Schofield T. Provider-Patient Communication, Patient-Centered Care, and the Mangle of Practice. Health Communication. 1997;9(1):27–43.
23. Lynn J, DeGrazia D. An outcomes model of medical decision making. Theor Med. 1991 Dec;12(4):325–43.
24. Robinson CA. Managing life with a chronic condition: the story of normalization. Qual Health Res. 1993 Feb;3(1):6–28.
25. Deatrick JA, Knafl KA, Murphy-Moore C. Clarifying the concept of normalization. Image—The Journal of Nursing Scholarship. 1999;31(3):209–14.
26. Chewning B, Sleath B. Medication decision-making and management: a client-centered model. Soc Sci Med. 1996 Feb;42(3):389–98.
27. Wagner EH, Austin BT, Von Korff M. Organizing care for patients with chronic illness. Milbank Q. 1996;74(4):511–44.
28. Stewart M, Brown JB, Donner A, McWhinney IR, Oates J, Weston WW, Jordan J. The impact of patient-centered care on outcomes. The Journal of Family Practice. 2000 Sep;49(9):796–804.
29. Bodenheimer T, Lorig K, Holman H, Grumbach K. Patient self-management of chronic disease in primary care. JAMA. 2002 Nov 20;288(19):2469–75.
30. Glasgow RE, Anderson RM. In diabetes care, moving from compliance to adherence is not enough. Something entirely different is needed. Diabetes Care. 1999 Dec;22(12):2090–2.
31. Lorig K, Holman H, Sobel D, Laurent D, Gonzalez V, Minor M. Living a healthy life with chronic conditions: self-management of heart disease, arthritis, diabetes, asthma, bronchitis, emphysema and others. Boulder, Colorado: Bull Publishing Company; 2000.
32. Allison MJ, Keller C. Self-efficacy intervention effect on physical activity in older adults. Western Journal of Nursing Research. 2004 Feb;26(1):31–46; discussion 47–58.

33. Luszczynska A, Gregajtys A, Abraham C. Effects of a self-efficacy intervention on initiation of recommended exercises in patients with spondylosis. Journal of Aging and Physical Activity. 2007 Jan;15(1):26–40.
34. Strecher VJ, DeVellis BM, Becker MH, Rosenstock IM. The role of self-efficacy in achieving health behavior change. Health Educ Q. 1986 Spring;13(1):73–92.
35. Bandura A. Self-efficacy: toward a unifying theory of behavioral change. Psychol Rev. 1977 Mar;84(2):191–215.
36. Roter DL, Hall JA, Merisca R, Nordstrom B, Cretin D, Svarstad B. Effectiveness of interventions to improve patient compliance: a meta-analysis. Med Care. 1998 Aug;36(8):1138–61.
37. van Eijken M, Tsang S, Wensing M, de Smet PA, Grol RP. Interventions to improve medication compliance in older patients living in the community: a systematic review of the literature. Drugs Aging. 2003;20(3):229–40.
38. DeBusk RF, Miller NH, Superko HR, Dennis CA, Thomas RJ, Lew HT, Berger WE, 3rd, Heller RS, Rompf J, Gee D, Kraemer HC, Bandura A, Ghandour G, Clark M, Shah RV, Fisher L, Taylor CB. A case-management system for coronary risk factor modification after acute myocardial infarction. Ann Intern Med. 1994 May 1;120(9):721–9.
39. Miller NH, Hill M, Kottke T, Ockene IS. The multilevel compliance challenge: recommendations for a call to action. A statement for health care professionals. Circulation. 1997 Feb 18;95(4):1085–90.
40. Peters AL, Davidson MB, Ossorio RC. Management of patients with diabetes by nurses with support of subspecialists. HMO Pract. 1995 Mar;9(1):8–13.
41. Safran DG, Wilson IB, Rogers WH, Montgomery JE, Chang H. Primary care quality in the Medicare Program: comparing the performance of Medicare health maintenance organizations and traditional fee-for-service medicare. Arch Intern Med. 2002 Apr 8;162(7):757–65.
42. Safran DG. Defining the future of primary care: what can we learn from patients? Ann Intern Med. 2003 Feb 4;138(3):248–55.
43. Murphy J, Chang H, Montgomery JE, Rogers WH, Safran DG. The quality of physician-patient relationships. Patients' experiences 1996–1999. J Fam Pract. 2001 Feb;50(2):123–9.
44. Safran DG, Rogers WH, Tarlov AR, Inui T, Taira DA, Montgomery JE, Ware JE, Slavin CP. Organizational and financial characteristics of health plans: are they related to primary care performance? Arch Intern Med. 2000 Jan 10;160(1):69–76.
45. Retchin SM, Brown B. Management of colorectal cancer in Medicare health maintenance organizations. J Gen Intern Med. 1990 Mar–Apr;5(2):110–4.
46. Forrest CB, Shi L, von Schrader S, Ng J. Managed care, primary care, and the patient-practitioner relationship. J Gen Intern Med. 2002 Apr;17(4):270–7.
47. Clement DG, Retchin SM, Brown RS, Stegall MH. Access and outcomes of elderly patients enrolled in managed care. JAMA. 1994 May 18;271(19):1487–92.
48. Roulidis ZC, Schulman KA. Physician communication in managed care organizations: opinions of primary care physicians. J Fam Pract. 1994 Nov;39(5):446–51.
49. Greenfield S, Kaplan S, Ware JE, Jr. Expanding patient involvement in care. Effects on patient outcomes. Ann Intern Med. 1985 Apr;102(4):520–8.
50. Guadagnoli E, Ward P. Patient participation in decision-making. Soc Sci Med. 1998 Aug;47(3):329–39.

51. Yach D, Hawkes C, Gould CL, Hofman KJ. The global burden of chronic diseases: overcoming impediments to prevention and control. JAMA. 2004 Jun 2;291(21):2616–22.
52. Cowen EL. The wooing of primary prevention. Am J Community Psychol. 1980 Jun;8(3):258–84.
53. Institute of Medicine. Crossing the Quality Chasm: A New Health System for the Twenty-first Century. Washington DC: National Academy Press; 2001.
54. Berry LL, Seiders K, Wilder SS. Innovations in access to care: a patient-centered approach. Ann Intern Med. 2003 Oct 7;139(7):568–74.
55. Adler NE, Newman K. Socioeconomic disparities in health: pathways and policies. Health Aff (Millwood). 2002 Mar–Apr;21(2):60–76.
56. Adler NE, Ostrove JM. Socioeconomic status and health: what we know and what we don't. Ann N Y Acad Sci. 1999;896:3–15.
57. Keppel KG. Ten Largest Racial and Ethnic Health Disparities in the United States based on Healthy People 2010 Objectives. Am J Epidemiol. 2007 Apr 26.
58. DeVoe JE, Fryer GE, Phillips R, Green L. Receipt of preventive care among adults: insurance status and usual source of care. Am J Public Health. 2003 May;93(5):786–91.
59. Ettner SL. The relationship between continuity of care and the health behaviors of patients: does having a usual physician make a difference? Med Care. 1999 Jun;37(6):547–55.
60. McGinnis JM. Investing in health: the role of disease prevention. In: Blank RH, Bonnicksen AL, editors. Emerging issues in biomedical policy: an annual review. Vol. 1. New York: Columbia University Press, 1992. p. 13–26.
61. Sickles EA. Mammography screening and the self-referred woman. Radiology. 1988 Jan;166(1 Pt 1):271–3.
62. Smedley BD, Stith AY, Nelson AR. Unequal Treatment: Confronting Racial and Ethnic Disparities in Health Care. Washington, DC: National Academy Press; 2002.
63. Piette JD, Wagner TH, Potter MB, Schillinger D. Health insurance status, cost-related medication underuse, and outcomes among diabetes patients in three systems of care. Med Care. 2004 Feb;42(2):102–9.

Index